SBAs for the Final FRCA

D1380760

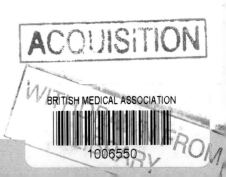

SBAs for the Final FRCA

Caroline Whymark
Consultant in Anaesthesia and Pain Medicine,
University Hospital Crosshouse,
NHS Ayrshire and Arran, UK

Ross Junkin
Consultant in Anaesthesia,
University Hospital Crosshouse,
NHS Ayrshire and Arran, UK

Judith Ramsey
Consultant in Anaesthesia and Intensive Care Medicine,
University Hospital Ayr,
NHS Ayrshire and Arran, UK

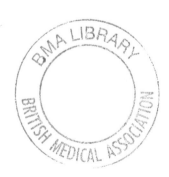

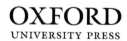

OXFORD
UNIVERSITY PRESS

OXFORD
UNIVERSITY PRESS

Great Clarendon Street, Oxford, OX2 6DP,
United Kingdom

Oxford University Press is a department of the University of Oxford.
It furthers the University's objective of excellence in research, scholarship,
and education by publishing worldwide. Oxford is a registered trade mark of
Oxford University Press in the UK and in certain other countries

© Oxford University Press 2019

The moral rights of the authors have been asserted

First Edition published in 2019
Impression: 1

Published in the United States of America by Oxford University Press
198 Madison Avenue, New York, NY 10016, United States of America

British Library Cataloguing in Publication Data

Data available

Library of Congress Control Number: 2018966985

ISBN 978–0–19–880329–4

Printed and bound by
CPI Group (UK) Ltd, Croydon, CR0 4YY

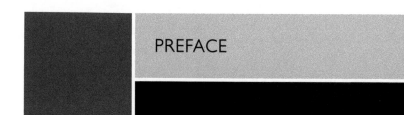

PREFACE

Good preparation is vital for success in the Final FRCA examination. Many candidates report that the SBA questions are the most difficult part of the exam in which to score well. Not only do they test advanced clinical decision making, but these questions are relatively new to postgraduate exams in Anaesthesia and therefore there are very few accurate examples available to inform exam preparation.

This book is designed to address that need and is written primarily as a formative tool to direct study. Candidates can be assured that the questions in this book reflect the breadth of the syllabus including subspecialties of which they may have limited experience. We include a mock exam chapter for completeness.

All questions in this book are original, and many are based on real scenarios we have encountered in our day-to-day practice, thus ensuring their clinical relevance. Each is fully explained and referenced. The book is closely linked to Intermediate Training under the 2010 Curriculum. Each chapter is dedicated to a specific unit of anaesthetic training. The book can therefore be used to consolidate studying on specific topics and identify knowledge gaps. The explanations and references direct the candidate to further learning resources.

We have a shared interest in medical education and are committed to delivering training of the highest standard. Together we developed and deliver a successful Final FRCA preparation course in the West of Scotland. Delegates consistently exceeded the national pass rates for this part of the exam.

We have used this experience and feedback from delegates to guide the creation of this book.

Caroline Whymark
Judith Ramsey
Ross Junkin

CONTENTS

List of abbreviations   ix

1 Introduction   1

2 Perioperative medicine
Questions   5
Answers   12

3 Trauma and orthopaedics
Questions   19
Answers   27

4 Resuscitation and transfer
Questions   35
Answers   43

5 ENT, maxillofacial, and ophthalmology
Questions   49
Answers   56

6 Vascular and general
Questions   63
Answers   70

7 Day surgery, preoperative assessment, gynaecology, urology, and plastics

Questions 77

Answers 84

8 Cardiothoracics

Questions 93

Answers 98

9 Neurosurgery

Questions 105

Answers 111

10 Paediatrics

Questions 117

Answers 123

11 Obstetrics

Questions 129

Answers 135

12 Intensive care

Questions 143

Answers 149

13 Chronic pain

Questions 155

Answers 160

14 Mock exam

Questions 167

Answers 175

Index 185

ABBREVIATIONS

ADP	adenosine diphosphate
ALS	advanced life support
ASA	aspirin
AV	atrioventricular
BMI	body mass index
BMS	bare metal stent
CABG	coronary artery bypass graft
CBG	capillary blood glucose
CEA	carotid endarterectomy
COPD	chronic obstructive pulmonary disease
CPET	cardiopulmonary exercise testing
CPR	cardiopulmonary resuscitation
CT	computed tomography
CVS	central venous catheter
DES	drug-eluting stent
DKA	diabetic ketoacidosis
DLCO	diffusing capacity of the lungs for carbon monoxide
ECG	electrocardiogram
EEG	electroencephalogram
ET	endotracheal
FBC	full blood count
FEV_1	forced expiratory volume in 1 second
FVC	forced vital capacity
GCS	Glasgow Coma Scale
GTN	glyceryl trinitrate
Hb	haemoglobin
IABP	intra-aortic balloon pump
ICU	intensive care unit
IPPV	intermittent positive pressure ventilation
IV	intravenously
LMA	laryngeal mask airway

MAC	minimum alveolar concentration
MAP	mean arterial pressure
MCH	mean corpuscular haemoglobin
MCV	mean corpuscular volume
MI	myocardial infarction
OIH	opioid-induced hyperalgesia
ORIF	open reduction and internal fixation
OSA	obstructive sleep apnoea
PBF	pulmonary blood flow
PCA	patient-controlled analgesia
PEA	pulseless electrical activity
PEEP	positive end-expiratory pressure
PEF	peak expiratory flow
PONV	postoperative nausea and vomiting
PTCA	percutaneous transluminal coronary angioplasty
PTE	pulmonary thromboembolism
PVR	pulmonary vascular resistance
RSI	rapid sequence induction
SAH	subarachnoid haemorrhage
SIADH	syndrome of inappropriate antidiuretic hormone secretion
ST	stent thrombosis
SVR	systemic vascular resistance
TAP	transabdominal plane
TIVA	total intravenous anaesthesia
TURP	transurethral resection of prostate
U&E	urea and electrolytes

chapter 1
INTRODUCTION

To pass the written part of the FRCA, candidates must achieve the pass mark for the SAQs and the MCQ/SBA papers combined. Therefore, doing particularly well in one paper, or one area, can compensate for another in which you have scored poorly.

The 30 SBA questions is an area that candidates commonly find difficult. There is a feeling these questions are unjust and that it is impossible to second guess the examiners and choose the correct option. They feel further punished that four marks are awarded for each correct answer or lost for an incorrect choice. While this reflects the fact that four answers have been eliminated in the course of choosing the best answer, candidates often state it is an unfair 'all or nothing' way to mark these questions. They can commonly narrow the choice down to a final two options but report finding it difficult to then choose between them. They receive no credit having successfully eliminated three of the options and cite the SBA element as being the reason they failed the examination.

These comments however are not supported by examination success data published by the RCoA. The pass rate for this paper was consistent at around 70% before and after the introduction of the SBA component in September 2011.

We believe the concepts behind the SBAs are misunderstood by many. When asked to write a SBA question, candidates inevitably produce a five-part A to E multiple choice question but with only one correct answer. The finer points of SBA questions are lost among quickly written revision aids containing what the authors believe to be examination standard questions, when often they are not. Further, because SBAs are a relatively new element to the FRCA there is a limited bank of questions, and a highly restricted number in the public domain. Both these factors make practice of these questions difficult.

Part of exam success is practice of the technique and question type in advance. We believe the practice of SBAs is an area to which candidates do not give enough attention.

In our experience, candidates practice SBA questions as a mock exam, attempting 30 questions covering an array of topics in the curriculum. This is evidenced by the many books that are written in this way. Candidates cannot wait to ditch the books and studying proper to try the mock exam and find out their score. As they mark their own paper, they try to learn from their mistakes and end up with a list of random facts that have popped up from the explanations.

Since 2014, the subject matter of the final FRCA SBA questions have changed from consisting of 15 questions from general training and 15 from specialty units of training to now closely follow and reflect the key units of training of the intermediate curriculum. All questions can be mapped to specific competences and all areas of the curriculum can be sampled. The result is less of an emphasis on general anaesthesia and more pointed inclusion of the other key units of training.

Learning is much more effective when achieved within context. It makes sense to practice questions which reflect the studying you have most recently done and with this book you can do this. The questions in each chapter pertain to one or two key units of training enabling candidates to study one area of the curriculum and then test their knowledge by attempting themed SBAs on that same unit of training. This makes practice questions much more of a formative tool as the explanations can highlight areas where specific knowledge is required and any additional points learned can be incorporated into that which was recently studied. This is much more effective way to test the quality of studying and retention of knowledge. Visiting a topic again in a different format such as this, reinforces learning and is much more useful than the traditional mixture of practice exam questions and summative scores.

Another reason for poor performance in the SBA section is the questions. That is not as silly as it sounds. Many candidates fall into the trap of immediately 'recognizing' the question. They assume it is identical to one they have seen before and do not bother to finish reading it accurately. Instead they go straight to the answers and choose the option they remember being correct the time before. Often it is not.

As well as questions published by the RCoA, there are many other 'remembered' questions: transcripts from peers who have already taken the exam. This practice is fraught with error and inaccuracies. The substitution of only a few words in the question can change the thrust of the question entirely. Questions can and do change in subtle ways and peers sitting the exam are not primarily focused on remembering the small print for someone else. It boils down to the simple fact of reading the question accurately and answering the question that is being asked, not the question you think is being asked or the one that was asked in a previous exam.

When new questions are constructed for the SBA paper, a great deal of attention and discussion takes place around the specific wording, to improve the clarity of the question and avoid ambiguity. No words are chosen by accident; each has been closely considered and discussed so the candidate must pay close attention to the words used, their meaning, and the reason for their use. There will be a specific reason that the patient is 69 years old (not 70) and had a myocardial infarction two months ago (not three) and needs an emergency operation (not an elective one). Usually a question is testing one piece of knowledge. Think about what that is from the detail provided in the question.

We have followed this practice when compiling this book of questions. No questions in this book are remembered from any exam, taken from websites, or indeed existed in the past. We have written de novo questions following the required structure and format. We have peer reviewed each question and have referenced our correct answers to justify them and have often added additional references which discuss the reasons other answers are less correct. In the nature of SBA's, a judgement must be made in providing a correct answer. Clearly there will be instances of differing opinion amongst readers given the often encountered clinical contention and we, the authors, are fully accepting of this fact. Hence we have simply provided what we believe is a "best answer" given the clinical scenario described. Any debate which this provokes will only add to the candidates ability to assess, scrutinise, balance and ultimately judge the information provided.

SBA technique

Questions for the examination itself are written to exacting standards and follow a set format. Rather than testing simple factual knowledge, SBAs test deduction, critical appraisal, and balancing of risks in an often complex clinical setting. Their aim is to assess *application* of knowledge within a *specific clinical context*, rather than to recall isolated facts. They focus on important concepts or significant clinical events. The SBAs are written very precisely to a template containing many rules. The stem, or introduction, consists of a vignette of clinical or laboratory information which can be up to 60 words in length. This will be followed by a short lead in to which the best answer must be chosen. The lead in should be a simple, direct question answerable by applying knowledge and information presented in the stem.

The five options are succinct and should each relate to a defined concept only. There should be no double options; 'Do X because of Y', instead it should be 'Do X'.

In SBA questions all five answers will be plausible. Several may also be possible. More than one or two answers may be correct or acceptable. But one option will be better than the others, and this is the answer. It is often the case that three options can be clearly eliminated and it is difficult to decide between the remaining two. There may be debate around the 'best' answers: some having a degree of subjectivity, and others reflecting true variations between the varied practice of different clinicians. At times, not all the examiners will agree on what the best answer ought to be. This makes it difficult for trainers and candidates to predict what specifically makes the best answer better than the others. The Royal College of Anaesthetists look for the answer they would expect to receive from a competent trainee anaesthetist transitioning into higher training. That is, one at the beginning of ST5 who is practising safely and who errs on the side of caution. Notably, the best answer is not that given by a Consultant with a niche role in the particular clinical area. It is also not the answer given by a very experienced Consultant who may know 'What works for me' and will draw on lengthy experience to aid clinical decision making.

When two correct options remain, candidates should choose the simplest one, the least invasive one, the one with the lowest risk to the patient. The safest one.

The first rule of answering these questions is to find your correct answer within the list of five options. To do so it is important not to colour your judgement by what you see listed there, because all the options may sound reasonable. Our advice is to firstly *cover* over all five options to the question. Next read the stem, and the lead in. Then STOP. Do not look at the options yet. Stop and think about the question, note the specific wording, decide what it is asking, and think about what you would actually do in your clinical practice when faced with this scenario. SBA questions are often written subsequent to real-life clinical dilemmas. If you do not know what you would do, think who you would ask to help you and what kind of help you require. Do you need help to decide between two options? Do you need help with a specific skill only? Or do you need help with the decision making? In case of the last one, try to imagine what your senior colleague would advise you to do if you telephoned them with this scenario. What if they were a Final examiner? What would they suggest you do? Once you have formulated what you believe to be the answer, only then uncover the options. If the answer you have arrived at is there, excellent! This is the one to select. Do not be tempted to change your mind to any of the distractors (incorrect answers). Congratulate yourself on having the self-discipline to cover the answers while you stop and think, because this is difficult to do.

If your answer is not listed then you have to use a different strategy. Try to eliminate as many wrong answers as you can. If you can eliminate four then that is fantastic. If, however, you can only eliminate three, you must apply the best guess strategy to the remaining two answers. When left with two options there is a 50% chance that any one person would guess correctly. Assuming you have some degree of knowledge relative to the question, your chances will be much closer to 100% than to 50%. You will not always choose correctly, nor will you agree that the correct answer is in fact the best one. That is the nature of these questions and there will always be some conflict of opinion. If you have prepared well and practised your technique, such guesses will be few and far between.

Remember to use this approach by thinking of the patient safety initiative, introduced to prevent inadvertent wrong-sided placement of peripheral nerve blocks: 'Stop Before You Block'. This asks you to stop and re-check the side, needle poised, immediately prior to its insertion into the skin. Apply the same technique in this paper. Immediately before reading the question, stop and cover the answers. You must *Stop Before You (Mentally) Block*.

Summary

We hope this book will be a helpful adjunct to studying for the FRCA, that it will help ensure the candidate covers the whole intermediate curriculum during their preparation, and provide a marker of the effectiveness of that studying. Importantly it will provide many opportunities for candidates to practice critical, accurate, and active question reading. We have provided suggested best answers which will no doubt provoke healthy debate amongst candidates around areas of established clinical contention and which will stand them in good stead when they take the real exam.

1. **Which of the options is most characteristic of a perioperative myocardial infarction?**
   A. Occurs intraoperatively
   B. Is associated with ST elevation
   C. The patient complains of shortness of breath and chest pain
   D. Has a mortality of up to 25%
   E. Occurs secondary to mismatched oxygen supply and demand

2. **Regarding the minimum standards of monitoring during anaesthesia and recovery, which of the following statements best reflects the most recent guidance?**
   A. The minimum standard of monitoring recommended varies with the seniority of the anaesthetist
   B. A processed electroencephalography (EEG) monitor is recommended when total intravenous anaesthesia (TIVA) with neuromuscular blockade is employed
   C. Temperature must be monitored during all cases
   D. The minimum standard of monitoring recommended varies depending on the clinical area
   E. If the minimum standards of monitoring cannot be met then anaesthesia should be postponed or cancelled

3. **A 78-year-old woman is listed for emergency laparotomy. She has presented with acute upper abdominal pain and a pneumoperitoneum is evident on chest X-ray. Her medical history includes early Alzheimer's disease and osteoarthritis. Drug history includes galantamine and diclofenac. The best plan regarding muscle relaxant use is:**
   A. Atracurium and wait for spontaneous inactivation
   B. Atracurium and neostigmine
   C. Rocuronium and sugammadex
   D. Rocuronium and neostigmine
   E. Suxamethonium

4. A 65-year-old man presents to preoperative assessment before elective inguinal hernia repair. He has no medical history and good exercise capacity. You are asked to review his electrocardiogram (ECG), which shows progressive prolongation of the PR interval culminating in a non-conducted P-wave on a repeating four-beat cycle. The most correct action now is:

    A. 24-hour ECG
    B. Echocardiography
    C. Check electrolytes
    D. Cardiopulmonary exercise testing
    E. No further investigation required

5. You are asked to review a postoperative patient in recovery. He is complaining of severe central crushing chest pain radiating down his left arm. He appears grey and clammy and is very distressed. Bedside ECG reveals 4-mm horizontal ST segment depression in leads V1–V3, upright T-waves, and a dominant R wave in V2. The coronary artery most likely to be implicated is:

    A. Posterior descending artery
    B. Right marginal artery
    C. Circumflex artery
    D. Left anterior descending
    E. Left marginal artery

6. You have used a bronchoscope during a difficult intubation. The best means of reprocessing the bronchoscope for use in another patient is:

    A. Pasteurization
    B. Chemical disinfection
    C. Decontamination
    D. Steam sterilization
    E. Chemical sterilization

7. You assess a 60-year-old man for umbilical hernia repair as a day case. His wife volunteers that he snores a lot during sleep. The most discriminating sole predictor of obstructive sleep apnoea (OSA) is:

    A. BMI >35
    B. Age >50
    C. Neck circumference ≥43 cm (17 inches)
    D. Hypertension
    E. Smoking

8. **A 75-year-old man presents for elective total knee replacement. He has well-controlled atrial fibrillation and is stable on rivaroxaban. His U&E are normal. He experienced significant postoperative nausea and vomiting after his last general anaesthetic and requests regional anaesthesia. What is the best course of action regarding his anticoagulation?**

   A. Continue rivaroxaban and proceed with general anaesthesia
   B. Stop rivaroxaban seven days before surgery
   C. Stop rivaroxaban the day before allowing 24 hours before spinal is performed
   D. Allow 36 hours between last rivaroxaban dose and performance of spinal anaesthesia
   E. Continue rivaroxaban and proceed with spinal anaesthesia

9. **A 36-year-old man requires laparoscopic colectomy for ulcerative colitis. He is to be managed in accordance with local enhanced recovery practices. The best way to provide postoperative analgesia to enhance recovery for this patient is:**

   A. Patient-controlled analgesia (PCA) morphine
   B. Thoracic epidural (local anaesthetic and fentanyl)
   C. Spinal (local anaesthetic and diamorphine)
   D. Wound catheter with lidocaine infusion
   E. Bilateral transabdominal plane (TAP) blocks

10. **A 60-year-old man presents for a right total hip replacement. He has Parkinson's disease for which he takes levodopa and ropinirole. Which of the following would be the best management plan perioperatively?**

    A. Stop his ropinirole but continue levodopa
    B. Continue both his medications until induction and recommence as soon as possible
    C. Withhold both his medications before surgery
    D. Convert oral regimen to a subcutaneous apomorphine infusion prior to surgery
    E. Convert oral regimen to transdermal rotigoline prior to surgery

11. **A 64-year-old man presents for renal stone fragmentation surgery under general anaesthesia. He has a pacemaker *in situ* for sick sinus syndrome. Which statement is the most accurate regarding pacemaker management perioperatively?**

    A. Lithotripsy is contraindicated
    B. Peripheral nerve stimulation should be avoided
    C. A magnet should be placed over the pacemaker during surgery
    D. Monopolar diathermy should be used in preference to bipolar diathermy
    E. Rate modulator function should be deactivated prior to surgery

12. **A 55-year-old man is day 2 post operation following repair of a large epigastric hernia. He is a smoker, has type 2 diabetes and chronic renal failure stage 3. He is using a morphine PCA and has good pain relief but complains of severe nausea. You decide to stop his morphine PCA and replace it with oral oxycodone. When compared with oral morphine, the benefit of oral oxycodone in this patient is:**
    A. It has more affinity for central mu receptors than peripheral
    B. It is safer in renal failure
    C. It does not require metabolism by cytochrome p450 CYP2D6
    D. It has a second mechanism of action by increasing noradrenaline (norepinephrine) and serotonin
    E. It is more potent than morphine

13. **A 60-year-old woman presents with a carcinoid tumour in her terminal ileum. She has been experiencing weight loss, flushing, sweating, and hypertension in the last six months. She is to have the tumour surgically removed. What would be the best medication to treat her symptoms preoperatively?**
    A. Phenoxybenzamine
    B. Doxazosin
    C. Methysergide
    D. Octreotide
    E. Aprotinin

14. **You assess a 71-year-old lady requiring a primary total hip replacement. She has a past medical history of hypertension. On examination you hear a loud ejection systolic murmur and arrange further investigation. What echocardiogram finding is most suggestive of severe aortic stenosis?**
    A. Mean gradient across aortic valve of 35 mmHg
    B. Peak gradient across aortic valve of 60 mmHg
    C. Aortic jet velocity of 3 m/s
    D. Valve area of 0.9 cm^2
    E. Presence of bicuspid aortic valve

15. **A 65-year-old lady presents for a total knee replacement. She has polymyalgia rheumatica and has been on 15 mg of prednisolone for the last nine months. What is the most appropriate perioperative management of her steroid use?**
    A. Continue usual oral dose of 15 mg daily
    B. Withhold oral dose and give 25 mg hydrocortisone intravenously (IV) at induction
    C. Give usual oral dose and 25 mg IV hydrocortisone at induction
    D. Give usual oral dose with 25 mg IV hydrocortisone at induction and continue 25 mg IV once daily for 48 hours postoperatively
    E. Give usual oral dose with 25 mg IV hydrocortisone at induction with 25 mg IV three to four times daily for 48 hours postoperatively

16. **An 89-year-old man is scheduled for laparoscopic sigmoid colectomy in two days' time. He has no cardiovascular or respiratory comorbidities. He does not smoke and denies drinking any alcohol. He weighs 54 kg, lives alone, and walks with the assistance of a stick. The best way to minimize the risk of postoperative delirium is:**

A. Ensuring that his hearing and visual aids are worn at all times
B. Sedation on the intensive treatment unit (ITU) postoperatively
C. Haloperidol 0.5–1 mg intramuscularly (IM) as required
D. Starting diazepam 2 mg orally as required preoperatively
E. Encourage naps during the day as required

17. **A 48-year-old man with a body mass index (BMI) of 51 is having bariatric surgery. You elected to perform an awake fibreoptic intubation. At the end of the procedure he is fully reversed using sugammadex with good tidal volumes and you have pre-oxygenated with 100% oxygen. He is cardiovascularly stable. What is the most appropriate plan for extubation?**

A. Deep extubation
B. Elective tracheostomy
C. Delay extubation and take to ICU for prolonged recovery
D. Awake extubation once obeying commands
E. Place an airway exchange catheter before extubating

18. **A 64-year-old man with chronic liver disease requires a right hemicolectomy for adenocarcinoma. Which is the best test to assess the synthetic function of his liver?**

A. Serum albumin
B. Serum bilirubin
C. Prothrombin time
D. Aspartate aminotransferase (AST)
E. Alanine aminotransferase (ALT)

19. **Which option best describes the information available on the label of packaged sterilized devices?**

A. Date of sterilization, sterilizer used, and identification of person who carried out sterilization
B. Date instruments used, cycle or load number (from sterilizer), expiration date of sterilization
C. Location of sterilizing service, sterilizer used, identification of person who carried out sterilization
D. Type of device, date of sterilization, log of number of times sterilized
E. Sterilizer used, cycle or load number (from sterilizer), date of sterilization

20. The Cochrane Collaboration provides guidance on the evidence base for medical practices. Which of the following best describes their approach to assessment of published research?
    A. A six-point scale is used
    B. Level 1 evidence is the least acceptable level of evidence
    C. Case reports count as Level 5 evidence
    D. The strongest evidence requires a published review of many well-designed randomized controlled trials
    E. Opinions of respected authorities are Level 4 evidence

21. Which of the following is the most likely to result in persistent contamination of a medical device following attempted sterilization?
    A. The use of steam as the method of sterilization
    B. The use of low-temperature sterilization
    C. Device being made of plastic
    D. Poor decontamination of device
    E. Poor disinfection of device

22. You review a 68-year-old man with weight loss and dyspnoea. You note he has a sodium level of 119 mmol/L. His medications are aspirin and amlodipine. He has no peripheral oedema. The results of his tests are as follows: potassium 4.3 mml/L, Urea 6.7 mmol/L, creatinine 74 µmol/L, serum osmolality 26 mOsmol/kg, urinary sodium 43 mmol/L, urine osmolality 230 mOsmol/kg. The most likely diagnosis is:
    A. Severe dehydration
    B. Syndrome of inappropriate antidiuretic hormone secretion (SIADH)
    C. Renal failure
    D. Water overload
    E. Heart failure

23. You anaesthetize a 56-year-old woman for rigid oesophagoscopy. She has no significant medical history. You extubate her awake and then notice that her upper front incisor has been completely avulsed. She has good dentition, no gum disease, and otherwise good oral hygiene. The best initial response is:
    A. Push the tooth back into the socket and hold for several minutes
    B. Discard the tooth
    C. Discuss with dentist
    D. Place the avulsed tooth in milk
    E. Place the avulsed tooth in sterile saline

24. **A 68-year-old man is scheduled for laparoscopic upper gastrointestinal surgery for carcinoma in two weeks time. His haemoglobin is 110 g/L and his ferritin is 25 µg/L. The best means of preoperative optimization is:**
    A. Give oral iron therapy
    B. Give intravenous iron
    C. Give two units of allogenic blood the night before surgery
    D. Give erythropoietin (EPO)
    E. Arrange pre-donation of autologous blood

25. **A 20-year-old male on an opioid substitution programme requires acute appendicectomy. He currently takes 30 mg of methadone each day. The best way to manage his acute pain in the perioperative period would be:**
    A. Continue usual 30 mg of methadone and give only non-opioid analgesics adjuncts
    B. Continue usual 30 mg of methadone and give additional short-acting parenteral opioids and non-opioid adjuncts
    C. Continue usual 30 mg of methadone and give PCA morphine postoperatively
    D. Stop methadone on day of surgery and give PCA morphine with background infusion postoperatively
    E. Stop methadone and convert to equivalent dose of MST, give sevredol in addition for acute pain

1. D

Perioperative myocardial infarction (MI) can be difficult to diagnose as it usually presents without the typical symptoms associated with myocardial ischaemia. Further, the abnormal physiological signs are common and can occur non-specifically in the perioperative setting.

Two types of MI can occur. Type 1 is due to rupture or fissuring of plaques in response to tachycardia and hypertension and is compounded by the surgery-conferred pro-coagulant pro-thrombotic state. Type 2 is associated with oxygen demand outstripping supply and pathological changes associated with both types are commonly found at post-mortem. Less than 2% of perioperative MIs are associated with ST elevation. The vast majority are preceded by a period of ST depression. Early mortality is high (as high as 25%) partly as there is no certainty over the best treatment in the perioperative phase. Beta-blockers are known to further increase mortality and the risks of antiplatelet and antithrombotic therapies are greater at this time. Proceeding to PCI is a complex decision in this period due to the requirement of dual antiplatelet therapy afterwards.

Reed-Poysden C, Gupta KJ. Acute coronary syndromes. *BJA Education* 2015; 15 (6): 286–293.

2. B

The guidelines published by the AAGBI in December 2015 state that the minimum standards of monitoring apply whenever and wherever general anaesthesia, regional anaesthesia, or sedation is given. If any required element is not available, it is up to the anaesthetist in charge to decide whether to proceed without it. If so, they must document why it was not available for use. Temperature should be monitored in cases lasting more than 30 min. It is recommended that the processed EEG should be used alongside TIVA and neuromuscular blockade. Data derived from it provide an additional source of information about the patient's condition but their efficacy in predicting awareness or predicting an adequate level of anaesthesia remains inconsistent and much debated.

Checketts MR, Alladi R, Ferguson K, et al. *Recommendations for Standards of Monitoring During Anaesthesia and Recovery.* London: Association of Anaesthetists of Great Britain and Ireland, 2015. Available at: http://onlinelibrary.wiley.com/doi/10.1111/anae.13316/full

3. C

Alzheimer's disease is associated with a loss of cholinergic neurons resulting in profound memory disturbances and irreversible impairment of cognitive function. Specific dementia treatment largely comprises the use of acetylcholinesterase inhibitors. Galantamine is one such drug. The anaesthetist should therefore be aware of the potential for interactions and consider avoiding neuromuscular blocking agents altogether. However, if muscle relaxation is required it should be noted that suxamethonium paralysis may be prolonged. Larger doses of non-depolarizing neuromuscular blocking agents may be required to achieve sufficient paralysis. Neostigmine may be relatively ineffective (due to already present cholinesterase inhibition). Larger doses of rocuronium can be given safely in the knowledge that reversal can be achieved predictably with sugammadex.

Alcorn S, Foo I. Perioperative management of patients with dementia. *BJA Education* 2017; 17 (3): 94–98.

4. E

The ECG finding is second-degree atrioventricular (AV) block, Mobitz type 1 (Wenckebach phenomenon). A serial lengthening of the PR interval occurs with consecutive beats culminating in a P-wave without a subsequent QRS before the cycle repeats itself. Mobitz type I is usually a benign rhythm, causing minimal haemodynamic disturbance and with low risk of progression to third degree (or complete) heart block. Asymptomatic patients with Mobitz type 1 rarely require treatment. Symptomatic patients usually respond to atropine. Permanent pacing is rarely required. The patient reports no specific cardiac symptoms and is having peripheral surgery. They can progress to surgery without delay for further investigation which is likely to be of low yield.

Mobitz type 2 is another form of second degree AV block which is at risk of deterioration to complete heart block. It describes intermittent non-conducted P-waves without progressive prolongation of the PR interval.

Hutchins D. Peri-operative cardiac arrhythmias: ventricular dysrhythmias. *Anaesthesia Tutorial of the Week* 2013; 285. Available at: https://www.aagbi.org/sites/default/files/285%20Perioperative%20 Cardiac%20Dysrhythmias%20-%20Part%202%20v2[1].pdf

5. A

The clinical presentation and ECG findings are consistent with a posterior myocardial infarction. The posterior wall is usually supplied by the posterior descending artery, a branch of the right coronary artery in 80% of individuals. The ECG findings provide a mirror/opposite of an anterior wall MI pattern. Thus, the lack of ST elevation in this condition means the diagnosis is often missed as ST elevation becomes ST depression, Q waves become R waves, and T waves remain upright. The posterior MI ECG is often held up to a light by the observer with the sheet turned back to front and upside down to reveal a classic ST elevation pattern through the paper, almost as if the ECG electrodes had been placed on the posterior chest.

Ramanathan T, Skinner H. Coronary blood flow: continuing education in anaesthesia. *Critical Care & Pain* 2005; 5 (2): 61–64.

6. B

Decontamination is removal of contaminants prior to disinfection or sterilization. Pasteurization uses hot water at 77 degrees for 30 min to achieve intermediate level disinfection. Sterilization processes render an object completely free of all microbial life but is a harsh enough process to damage various reusable medical equipment such as bronchoscopes. Chemical disinfection with 2% glutaraldehyde is commonly used to disinfect scopes after decontamination.

Sabir N, RamachandraV. Decontamination of anaesthetic equipment. *Continuing Education in Anaesthesia, Critical Care & Pain* 2004; 4. (4).

7. C

All the answers represent criteria often assessed during obstructive sleep apnoea (OSA) risk scoring such as in the STOP-BANG criteria. This is a mixture of patient questions and demographics as follows:

- Snoring?—do you snore loudly, e.g. to be heard through closed doors?
- Tired?—do you often feel tired or sleepy during daytime?

- · Observed—has anyone observed you stopping breathing, choking, or gasping during sleep?
- · Pressure—do you have high blood pressure?
- · BMI >35
- · Age >50 years
- · Neck circumference >43 cm (male) or >41 cm (female)
- · Gender = male?

Copyright © 2014 University Health Network, Toronto, Canada. This tool is presented for educational purposes and not to be used for screening patients.

Each question scores a point and grades risk of OSA as low (0–2), intermediate (3–4), or high (5–8). Increased scoring during STOP-BANG should prompt consideration of further screening tools such as the Epworth Sleepiness Scale (ESS) or indeed investigation with sleep studies. While the most common risk factor for OSA is obesity, the OSA tendency correlates best with increased neck circumference.

Williams JM, Hanning CD. Obstructive sleep apnoea. *British Journal of Anaesthesia CEPD Reviews* 2003; 3 (3): 69–74.

8. C

Rivaroxaban inhibits platelet aggregation induced by Factor Xa. It is used alone and in combination with other drugs to prevent thrombus formation in those at risk of embolic stroke and as treatment for VTE. There is no reversal agent available. Such newer anticoagulants have led to adjustments in the interval between discontinuation of the drugs and performance of neuraxial procedures, based on the degree of risk of thrombosis. Research has focussed on the pharmacokinetics of the drug and its effect on anticoagulant parameters by laboratory monitoring. It is recommended that waiting for at least two half-lives to elapse is an adequate balance between the coagulation risks of stopping treatment and the bleeding risk of developing a spinal haematoma. Half-life is commonly prolonged in the elderly and for rivaroxaban is 7–11 hours so double would be 22 hours. Platelet count is unchanged with this drug and coagulation studies may not be helpful. Risk is further minimized by avoiding multiple injection attempts, avoiding epidural catheter placement, and waiting for a period of one half-life minus time to peak plasma concentration before restarting treatment.

Benzon HT, Avram MJ, Green D, Bonow RO. New anti-coagulants and regional anaesthesia. *British Journal of Anaesthesia* 2013; 111 (suppl 1): i96–i113.

9. C

Enhanced recovery after surgery (ERAS) is a multidisciplinary and multimodal treatment package delivered in the perioperative period to reduce postoperative morbidity and length of stay in hospital by expediting return to normal physiology and function. One aspect of this is providing effective analgesia with minimal detrimental effects. Systemic opioids should be minimised where possible as this slows return of gut function and necessitates the patient being connected to an intravenous line. Epidural analgesia, particularly thoracic, is the preferred analgesia regimen for open abdominal surgery but the risk/benefit ratio for laparoscopic surgery is different and epidural analgesia is generally not required. Wound catheters work well in open surgery but their role is limited in laparoscopic surgery. TAP blocks are useful adjuncts but will not attenuate the stress response intraoperatively and are unlikely to provide sufficient analgesia alone.

Boulind CE, Ewings P, Bulley SH, et al. Feasibility study of analgesia via epidural versus continuous wound infusion after laparoscopic colorectal surgery. *British Journal of Surgery* 2013; 100: 395–402.

Jones NL, Edmonds L, Ghosh S, et al. A review of enhanced recovery for thoracic anaesthesia surgery. *British Journal of Anaesthesia* 2013; 68 (2): 179–189.

Levy BF, Scott MJ, Fawcett W, et al. Randomised clinical trial of epidural, spinal or PCA for patients undergoing laparoscopic colorectal surgery. *British Journal of Surgery* 2011; 98: 1068–1078.

10. B

Although antiparkinsonian medications can interfere with many anaesthetic drugs their withdrawal can result in severe relapse of symptoms therefore it is very important that the usual antiparkinsonian medications continue with minimum disruption. This patient should have all their usual preoperative doses and should be able to eat and drink very soon after surgery. There would be no need to add in anything else. They should be able to resume their oral regimen quickly so careful assessment and management of postoperative nausea and vomiting is recommended. Avoidance of dopamine antagonist antiemetic drugs (e.g. metoclopramide) is of paramount importance given the directly opposing action on the dopamine agonist Parkinsonian treatments. For patients who may not be able to manage anything orally or via the nasogastric route, e.g. if requiring emergency intra-abdominal surgery, conversion to apomorphine or rotigotine may be considered.

Chambers DJ, Sebastian J, Ahearn DJ. Parkinson's disease. *BJA Education* 2017; 17 (4): 145–149.

11. E

If a pacemaker has a rate modulator function this should be deactivated prior to surgery. Lithotripsy is safe provided the lithotripter is >6 inches away from the pacemaker device. Peripheral nerve stimulators are again considered safe provided they are used a safe distance from the pacemaker and not in a parallel axis with the pacemaker. A magnet should not now be placed over a pacemaker during surgery. They have unpredictable effects on the programming in modern pacemakers. Bipolar is the preferred diathermy used.

Diprose P, Pierce JMT. Anaesthesia for patients with pacemakers and similar devices. *Continuing Education in Anaesthesia, Critical Care & Pain* 2001; 11 (6): 166–170.

12. B

Oxycodone is a semi synthetic opioid that is commonly used in the postoperative period due to its superior side effect profile when compared with morphine. It has a potency twice that of morphine and hence increased affinity for all receptors. This is relevant when converting from one to the other and to be aware that the potential for addiction to opioid drugs is greater with those of higher potency and faster onset. Hence answer E is true but does not confer any benefit as pain is well controlled, so it is not the best answer. There is no central versus peripheral preference to its receptor binding but in the central nervous system (CNS) its action is greatest at supraspinal levels; hence oxycodone is not suited to intrathecal or epidural use.

Oxycodone works only at opioid receptors mu, kappa, and delta. It does not influence noradrenergic or seretonergic pathways. This is a feature of tramadol and tapentadol.

When taken orally its absorption and distribution kinetics are similar to morphine however the bioavailability is almost double: 70–80% compared with 30%. It is metabolized by hepatic enzymes, and phase 1 metabolism is dependent upon the cytochrome p450 pathway. The main enzyme responsible for metabolism of oxycodone is cytochrome P450 3A4. This enzyme is inhibited by many drugs including other opioids but is not subject to the pharmacogenetic variability of CYP2D6. This enzyme is important in the metabolism and conversion of code in to its active form, norcodeine.

The metabolites of oxycodone have only a fraction of the activity of the parent compound and do not accumulate in renal failure as is a significant risk with morphine and its metabolite M6G.

Holmquist GL. Opioid metabolism and effects of cytochrome p450. *Pain Medicine* 2009 (suppl 1) 10: S1-2009. Available at: https://nam01.safelinks.protection.outlook.com/ ?url=https%3A%2F%2Facademic.oup.com%2Fpainmedicine%2Farticle-abstract%2F10%2Fsuppl_1%2F S20%2F1914905&data=02%7C01%7C%7Cbb97b7cd6408412e156108d5a69b885c%7C84df9e7fe9f 640afb435aaaaaaaaaaaa%7C1%7C0%7C636598109299130468&sdata=LWAuuL4IC6mNCqeLFMUT SN%2F4S%2BfOvd172RVpuwLVhYw%3D&reserved=0

13. D

Carcinoid syndrome, although rare, can create serious problems to the anaesthetist, both by the nature and variability of clinical manifestations and by the complications that can occur perioperatively. Carcinoid tumours are rare, slow-growing neoplasms of neuroendocrine tissues. The classification of carcinoid tumours is based on the histological characteristics and site of origin which includes lung, stomach, and small and large intestine. As a group, carcinoid tumours represent a wide spectrum of neuroendocrine cell types including enterochromaffin or Kulchitsky cells, which have the potential to metastasize. The cells typically contain numerous membrane-bound neurosecretory granules composed of hormones and amines. The most familiar of these is serotonin, which is metabolized from its precursor, 5-hydroxytryptophan by a decarboxylase enzyme. The mediators released from these tumours when bypassing the hepatic metabolism, can lead to the possible development of carcinoid syndrome. This is a life-threatening complication potentially seen as a carcinoid crisis, which can lead to profound haemodynamic instability, flushing, and bronchospasm especially in a perioperative period. The use of octreotide, a synthetic analogue of somatostatin, has significantly reduced the perioperative morbidity and mortality. All these agents in the question answer are potential treatments but octreotide is considered the first-line agent.

Powell B, Al Mukhtar A, Mills GH. Carcinoid: the disease and its implications for anaesthesia. *Continuing Education in Anaesthesia, Critical Care & Pain* 2011; 11(1): 9–13.

14. D

The presence of a bicuspid valve is not one of the criteria included in grading of aortic stenosis. All the other measurements indicate moderate aortic stenosis except for a valve area of 0.9 cm squared. Peak gradient across the valve would be >65 mmHg, and mean gradient would be >40 mmHg in severe stenosis. Guidance on echocardiography-based quantification of aortic stenosis can be found in the ACA/AHA guidelines (and Bonow et al.).

Bonow R, Carabello B, Chatterjee K. American College of Cardiology/American Heart Association (ACC/AHA). 2006 guidelines for the management of patients with valvular heart disease. *Circulation* 2006; 114: e84–e231.

Bonow RO, Carabello BA, Chatterjee K, et al. Focused update practice incorporated into the ACC/ AHA 2006 guidelines for the management of patients with valvular heart disease. A report of the American College of Cardiology/American Heart Association Task Force on Practice Guidelines. *Circulation* 2008; 118: e523–661.

Chacko M, Weinberg L. Aortic valve stenosis: perioperative anaesthetic implications of surgical replacement and minimally invasive interventions. *Continuing Education in Anaesthesia, Critical Care & Pain* 2012; 12 (6): 295–301.

15. E

Most hospitals and trusts have guidelines for supplementation with hydrocortisone for patients on long-term corticosteroid therapy based on whether surgery is minor, moderate, or major. If the patient has been on more than 10 mg of prednisolone a day for more than three months they require their usual dose plus 100 mg/day for two to three days after major surgery.

Nicholson G, Burrin JM, Hall GM. Peri-operative steroid supplementation. *Anaesthesia* 1998; 53: 1091–1104.

16. A

Good basic care is the most important way to reduce the incidence of postoperative delirium. This includes glasses being worn, hearing aids being worn and working, being orientated to surroundings, visits from friends and family. Ensuring a regular diurnal sleep–wake pattern to allow a long, uninterrupted nocturnal sleep is preferable and short daytime naps should be avoided. Long hospital stays and admission to ITU worsen the condition. Haloperidol is seen as a last resort for rescue rather than prevention. Diazepam may be indicated if regular alcohol excess is suspected but should not be used routinely.

Deiner S, Silverstein JH. Postoperative delirium and cognitive dysfunction. *British Journal of Anaesthesia* 2009; 103 (1): i41–i46.

17. D

All are possible extubation plans, but D is the most appropriate as the patient is fully reversed, stable, and pre-oxygenated.

Popat M, Dravid R, Patel A, et al; Difficult Airway Society Extubation Guidelines Group. Difficult airway society for the management of tracheal extubation. *Anaesthesia* 2012; 67 (3): 318–340.

18. C

Synthetic liver function is best assessed by prothrombin time and it is used as a prognostic indicator in acute liver failure and after surgery in patients with chronic liver disease. The prothrombin time produced is a result of the appropriate synthesis of multiple clotting factors by the liver at different levels of the coagulation cascade. Albumin levels can also be a useful indicator in addition to the prothrombin time. Bilirubin levels are often elevated and the pattern of AST and ALT enzyme rise varies with the aetiology.

Vaja R, McNicol L, Sisley I. Anaesthesia for patients with liver disease. *Continuing Education in Anaesthesia, Critical Care & Pain* 2010; 10 (1): 15–19.

19. E

The sterilizer and load number is important in case a problem is detected and other potentially contaminated items need to be identified. The date the instruments were used is not relevant. Only some pieces of equipment have an expiry date on their sterilization status.

Ref e-LA Module 07d: core training basic sciences equipment.

20. D

A five-point scale with Levels I–V is used where I is the strongest evidence and V is the weakest level of evidence considered. This includes reports from expert committees and opinions of respected authorities. Case reports are not robust enough to enter the assessment process.

Cochrane. Available at: http://www.cochrane.org

21. D

Decontamination is the initial process required to remove the particulate matter from any device. Failure to do so prevents the sterilizing method making contact with the whole of the instrument and therefore cannot be sterilized entirely.

Ref e-LA Module 07d: core training basic sciences equipment.

22. B

SIADH fits the biochemical and clinical picture. Criteria for diagnosing SIADH include clinical euvolaemia, serum osmolality <275 mOmol/L, urine osmolality >100 mOsmol/L, urinary sodium >30 mmol/L, normal thyroid and adrenal function, and no recent diuretic use. In this case, the symptoms suggest SIADH secondary to bronchial carcinoma.

Hirst C, Allahabadiah A, Cosgrove J. The adult patient with hyponatraemia. *BJA Education* 2014; 15 (5): 248–252.

23. A

The root surfaces should not be touched before pushing it back into the socket. It should be expedited so that the dental ligament does not become dehydrated. Only replace an adult tooth from a healthy mouth, in a patient who is not immunocompromised. Risks and benefits of replacing a loose tooth in an asleep anaesthetized patient should be considered, as it could potentially behave as a foreign body in the airway. This patient is awake however. The injury should then be referred to a dentist for splinting. If the anaesthetist does not feel comfortable replacing the tooth, it can be stored in saline or milk pending dental review.

Paolinelis G, Renton T, Djemal S, et al. Dental trauma during anaesthesia. Safe Anaesthesia Liaison Group. 2012, National Patient Safety Agency. Available at: https://www.rcoa.ac.uk/system/files/CSQ-DentalTrauma.pdf.

24. B

Haemoglobin levels below 130 g/L in a man, or 120 g/L in a women (WHO 1968), should be improved preoperatively. A ferritin of <30 μg/L indicates severe iron deficiency. Oral iron is indicated if the surgery is non-urgent but treatment of gastric carcinoma should not be delayed for this reason. Intravenous iron is indicated to increase haemoglobin in the short term and reduce the risk of perioperative allogenic transfusion and the associated poorer outcomes in cancer surgery.

Kotze A, Harris A, Maker C, et al. British Committee for Standards in Haematology Guidelines on the identification and management of pre-operative anaemia. *British Journal of Haematology* 2015; 171 (3): 322–331.

25. B

Patients on daily doses of methadone can present a challenge when managing their acute pain in the perioperative period. They have tolerance to opioids and are relatively resistant to them meaning they may require seemingly large doses to achieve any effect. Their dependence on these drugs mean they are frightened and anxious about the continued supply of their methadone while in hospital. Some fear having additional opioid analgesia will rekindle their addictive tendency and cause them to default from their substitution therapy programme. Further, there can be a reluctance by medical and nursing staff to provide additional opioid analgesia. Best practice is to continue the usual dose of methadone throughout the perioperative period (assuming the gut is working) and to treat acute pain with fast acting, short duration parenteral opioids as required. Paracetamol and non-steroidal analgesics should be prescribed regularly.

Quinlan J, Cox F. Acute pain management in patients with drug dependence syndrome. International Association for the Study of Pain (IASP). *Pain Clinical Update* 2017; XXV: 1–8.

1. You see a patient two days following left total knee replacement. He complains of right foot drop since surgery. He had a spinal anaesthetic and wonders if this was the cause, although no complications were reported at the time. He is otherwise well and clinical examination confirms weak dorsiflexion of his right foot. What is the most likely cause?

   A. Cerebrovascular accident
   B. Poor intraoperative positioning and padding
   C. Spinal abscess
   D. Spinal haematoma
   E. Spinal nerve root injury

2. A frail 86-year-old female requires neck of femur fixation surgery. Her BMI is 18. Her core temperature is 36.1°C prior to induction of anaesthesia. Which process will be responsible for the largest amount of heat loss during anaesthesia and surgery?

   A. Radiation
   B. Convection
   C. Respiration
   D. Evaporation
   E. Conduction

3. A 67-year-old man completed a 2-unit blood transfusion during his revision hip arthroplasty 8 hours ago. He has developed a fever, urticarial rash, and back pain. His heart rate is 132, BP 95/50, respiratory rate is 32. He has passed 130 mL of very dark urine since surgery. His post-transfusion blood results show a haemoglobin level of 75 g/L. What is the most likely explanation for his deterioration?

   A. Transfusion-related acute lung injury
   B. Transfusion-associated circulatory overload
   C. Transfusion-associated graft versus host disease
   D. Transfusion-related bacterial infection
   E. Acute haemolytic transfusion reaction

4. **A 28-year-old woman presents with a trimalleolar fracture of her left ankle. She is haemodynamically stable. She is 27 weeks pregnant. She has had an uneventful pregnancy so far and has no other past medical history. What would be the most appropriate anaesthetic management?**

    A. Recommend conservative management of the fracture until 3rd trimester
    B. General anaesthesia with a laryngeal mask airway (LMA) *in situ*
    C. General anaesthesia and intubation without a rapid sequence induction
    D. General anaesthesia and intubation with a rapid sequence induction
    E. Spinal anaesthesia

5. **A 59-year-old woman had an elective total knee replacement earlier today under spinal block which included 0.2 mg of preservative-free morphine. She is now complaining of severe itch around her neck and chest. She is otherwise well. What would be the most effective treatment for her symptoms?**

    A. Chlorpheniramine
    B. Diclofenac
    C. Hydrocortisone
    D. Naltrexone
    E. Ondansetron

6. **A 72-year-old man is listed for an elective total hip replacement. Which of the following is the strongest indication for the use of perioperative cell salvage?**

    A. Preoperative haemoglobin level of 13 g/dL
    B. Preoperative ferritin level of 150 ng/L
    C. Von Willebrand's disease type 3
    D. 75 mg of aspirin stopped five days ago
    E. Anticipated blood loss of 500 mL

7. **A 79-year-old female who sustained a fractured neck of femur the previous day is scheduled for operative fixation with a dynamic hip screw. She has a past medical history of type 2 diabetes mellitus on metformin. She denies any history of chest pain, breathlessness, or syncope. Which of the following is most likely to result in postponement of surgery?**

    A. A loud ejection systolic murmur on auscultation
    B. Blood tests show urea 8.0 mmol/L and creatinine 158 mmol/L
    C. Fasting blood glucose this morning was 16 mmol/L
    D. ECG (electrocardiogram) shows atrial fibrillation with rate of 92 bpm
    E. SpO$_2$ 96% on 2 L/min oxygen, RR 18 breaths/min. Apyrexial

8. **You anaesthetize a 34-year-old man for an open reduction and internal fixation (ORIF) of scaphoid fracture under general anaesthesia. You perform an ultrasound-guided radial nerve block above the elbow as part of your analgesia plan. Which is the most accurate statement regarding the performance of this block using ultrasound?**
   A. A high-frequency curvilinear probe provides the best images
   B. A reduced concentration of local anaesthetic is likely to be needed compared with the landmark technique
   C. The radial nerve appears hypo-echoic
   D. The probe should be orientated to show the nerve in the short axis
   E. Use of ultrasound removes risk of intravascular injection of local anaesthetic

9. **A 70-year-old lady is listed for a left dynamic hip screw for fixation of her fractured neck of femur. Her medical history includes hypothyroidism, hypertension, and depression. Her medication includes levothyroxine, bendroflumethazide, amlodipine, and phenelzine. You administer a spinal anaesthetic and 5 min later her heart rate decreases to 57 bpm and her blood pressure drops to 85/46 mmHg despite 500 mL of Hartmann's solution. What is the most appropriate drug to improve her cardiovascular status?**
   A. Phenylephrine
   B. Metaraminol
   C. Adrenaline (epinephrine)
   D. Noradrenaline (norepinephrine)
   E. Ephedrine

10. **A 48-year-old woman presents with severe pain, swelling, and erythema of her left forearm. The only history of trauma is of a small scratch while gardening a week ago. Her C-reactive protein (CRP) is 198, her white cell count (WCC) is 28, and her creatinine level is 180 µg/L. What is the gold standard method to confirm/refute necrotizing fasciitis as the diagnosis?**
    A. Blood cultures
    B. Computed tomography scan
    C. Percutaneous needle aspiration
    D. Surgical exploration and tissue biopsy
    E. Creatinine kinase level

11. **A 76-year-old lady is on the trauma list this morning for a femoral nailing. Her past medical history includes severe dementia, stable angina, and hypothyroidism. Her haemoglobin is 98 g/L. You notice in the orthopaedic a single sentence stating the patient is a Jehovah's witness. What is the best way to proceed?**

A. Postpone operation until you can speak to her next of kin to see what blood products they will permit

B. Proceed with a general anaesthetic and femoral nerve block. Give tranexamic acid and avoid transfusion of blood products even if life-threatening haemorrhage

C. Proceed with a general anaesthetic and femoral nerve block. Give tranexamic acid but use blood products if required to save her life as an Adults with Incapacity form is signed

D. Postpone operation until you speak to relatives and verify what her wishes would be in the event of life-threatening haemorrhage

E. Continue with spinal anaesthesia and femoral nerve block. Give tranexamic acid and avoid blood products even in life-threatening haemorrhage

12. **A 68-year-old man has sustained a hip fracture. He is listed for hemiarthroplasty. There are no other injuries apparent. He has stable angina and no other significant medical history. His resting ECG is normal. His full blood count reveals a haemoglobin of 10.9 g/dL. The most appropriate management is:**

A. Preoperative transfusion 1 unit packed red cells

B. Preoperative transfusion 2 units packed red cells

C. Crossmatch 2 units packed red cells and proceed

D. Crossmatch 4 units packed red cells and proceed

E. Grouped sample and proceed

13. **A 68-year-old man presents to hospital two weeks after elective right primary total hip replacement performed under uncomplicated spinal anaesthesia. He had complained of left thigh pain during his hospital admission but was reassured and sent home. He now reports left-sided reduced sensation in his lateral thigh skin with an unpleasant burning sensation. Neurological examination is otherwise normal. The most likely cause is:**

A. Meralgia paraesthetica

B. Soft tissue thigh injury

C. Conus injection

D. Compartment syndrome

E. Epidural haematoma

14. **A 68-year-old man presents to the Emergency Department having fallen. A chest X-ray shows three fractured ribs on his left side. He is Glasgow Coma Scale 15 with no other injury. He has well-controlled hypertension and mild angina. His pain has been controlled after titration of 0.1 mg/kg intravenous morphine and 1 g of paracetamol. His dynamic pain score is now 1. What would be the most appropriate initial pain management plan?**

    A. Regular paracetamol
    B. Insert a thoracic epidural
    C. Insert a left paravertebral catheter
    D. Morphine sulphate slow-release tablets twice a day with oramorph for breakthrough and regular paracetamol
    E. An intravenous morphine patient-controlled anaesthesia with regular paracetamol

15. **When considering risk of systemic local anaesthetic toxicity, which site for a regional block carries the highest risk?**

    A. Brachial plexus
    B. Intercostal
    C. Caudal
    D. Epidural
    E. Femoral

16. **You assess a 77-year-old man for excision of palmar Dupuytren's contracture. He is breathless at rest and uses home oxygen. His operation is necessary to allow him to use a zimmer frame to mobilize around his home. The best regional block to perform for the procedure is:**

    A. Median and ulnar nerve blocks at the wrist
    B. Median and ulnar nerve blocks at the antecubital fossa
    C. Axillary plexus block
    D. Supraclavicular block
    E. Interscalene block

17. **A 24-year-old male presents for a right knee arthroscopy and medial meniscectomy under general anaesthetic in day surgery. He is otherwise fit and well. What would be the best regional technique to use in addition to the general anaesthetic?**

    A. Psoas compartment block
    B. Adductor canal block
    C. Femoral block
    D. Sciatic nerve block
    E. Wound infiltration by the surgeon

18. **An 80-year-old woman is booked on the trauma list having fallen 24 hours previously causing a fracture of her neck of femur. She remains in significant pain. She gives a history of blackouts preceded by light-headedness over the last three months. Past medical history includes hypertension treated with lisinopril and bisoprolol. Heart sounds are normal and chest is clear. ECG today reveals normal sinus rhythm, rate 75 and normal axis. The most appropriate course of action is:**

   A. Postpone the operation pending investigation of blackouts
   B. Cancel the operation and advise conservative management of fracture
   C. Proceed to operation and plan for general anaesthesia
   D. Proceed to operation and plan for spinal anaesthesia
   E. Withhold bisoprolol, proceed to operation and plan for general anaesthesia

19. **A 74-year-old male is having a cemented hip hemiarthroplasty under spinal block. He has stable angina and chronic obstructive pulmonary disease. Two minutes after insertion of the prosthesis his oxygen saturations drop to 80% on 4 L of oxygen via a Hudson mask. He loses consciousness and his blood pressure is now 60/32 mmHg having previously been stable. Which of the following best describes the initial physiological cause of this clinical syndrome?**

   A. Decreased pulmonary artery pressure
   B. Increased systemic vascular resistance
   C. Increased central venous pressure
   D. Increased pulmonary vascular resistance
   E. Deceased systemic vascular resistance

20. **You anaesthetize a 63-year-old woman for manipulation of distal radial fracture. She is spontaneously ventilating on a laryngeal mask airway (LMA), breathing oxygen/air/sevoflurane to a minimum alveolar concentration (MAC) value of 1.0. On manipulation of the forearm she develops noisy breathing on inspiration. What is the most appropriate immediate action?**

   A. Increase sevoflurane to 8%
   B. 100% oxygen
   C. IV propofol
   D. IV rocuronium
   E. Remove LMA

21. **A 28-year-old professional rugby player has undergone rotator cuff repair. You administer general anaesthesia including 10 mg of morphine and an interscalene block. In recovery he reports a sensation of difficulty breathing. His respiratory rate is 18, oxygen saturation 97% on 4 L via a Hudson mask, and nerve stimulation shows he has four twitches with no detectable fade. The most likely cause of his breathing difficulty is:**
    A. Inadequate reversal
    B. Relative overdose of morphine
    C. Covert use of anabolic steroids
    D. Phrenic nerve palsy
    E. Anxiety

22. **An 84-year-old woman presents to the emergency department with a suspected fractured neck of femur. She had a simple fall on the way to the bathroom in her nursing home and it is 4 am. She has had 10 mg of morphine IM by the paramedics and a further 10 mg titrated IV since she arrived. She reports an ongoing pain score of 10/10 and the orthopaedic doctor has asked for your pain advice. The best management of her analgesia is:**
    A. Take to theatre for operative fixation
    B. Continue to titrate IV opioid
    C. Offer N_2O/O_2
    D. Administer oral ibuprofen and paracetamol
    E. Perform a femoral nerve block

23. **A 25-year-old man is admitted with a right compound mid-shaft tibial and fibular fracture following a simple fall. He is planned for operative fixation the next morning. He has a past medical history of deep venous thrombosis (DVT) five years ago following a hernia repair. He is on no regular medication. Overnight, he complains of severe right-sided leg pain and tingling. On examination, his leg is warm, tender, and swollen. The pedal pulse is faint. The wound dressing is dry. On examination, HR 105 bpm, regular, BP 110/65, RR 20, SaO_2 94% on 2 L of O_2 and temperature is 37.4°C. The most likely diagnosis is:**
    A. Deep vein thrombosis
    B. Compartment syndrome
    C. Cellulitis
    D. Necrotizing fasciitis
    E. Acute limb ischaemia

24. **A 68-year-old female with rheumatoid arthritis presents for a left shoulder hemiarthroplasty. She takes etoricoxib and methotrexate as treatment. You notice an abnormality on her cervical spine X-ray. What is the most common cervical spine abnormality associated with rheumatoid arthritis?**

    A. Atlanto-axial dislocation
    B. Anterior atlanto-axial subluxation
    C. Lateral atlanto-axial subluxation
    D. Sub-axial dislocation
    E. Sub-axial subluxation

25. **A 54-year-old presents for an ORIF of a fractured wrist. He has no major comorbidities. However, he is a heavy smoker with a chronic productive cough. He is being sent home to come in fasted for his operation tomorrow. You advise him on smoking cessation as part of your pre-assessment. What effect would be most likely if he stops smoking for 24 hours?**

    A. No effect
    B. Increased oxygen carriage by the blood
    C. Less reactive airways
    D. Reduced sputum production
    E. Reduced likelihood of postoperative respiratory failure

1. B

Postoperative complications may result from surgical, anaesthetic, or non-medical factors including patient positioning. Intraoperative positioning and padding may lead to prolonged pressure on the common peroneal nerve during anaesthesia which is a well-documented cause of postoperative foot drop. One must ensure adequate padding around the fibular head when positioning patients under general or regional anaesthesia for long periods of time. A central neurological cause is unlikely to cause such well-defined peripheral nerve lesions and in any case is very rare. Treatment is conservative and the transient neuropraxia will usually pass. However, the patient should also be counselled of the possibility that this may be a permanent injury.

Sawyer RJ, Richmond MN, Hickey JD, Jarrratt J. Peripheral nerve injuries associated with anaesthesia. *Anaesthesia* 2000; 55: 980–991.

2. A

These five mechanisms all contribute to heat loss from the body. Around 40% is estimated to be by radiation which is the largest.

Sullivan F, Edmondson C. Heat and temperature. *Continuing Education in Anaesthesia Critical Care & Pain* 2008; 8 (3): 104–107.

3. E

Acute haemolytic transfusion reactions present within 24 hours after a transfusion of ABO-incompatible red blood cells. Antigens on the donor red cells react with antibodies in the recipient's plasma leading to degranulation of mast cells, inflammation, increased vascular permeability, and hypotension. Intravascular haemolysis can occur leading to disseminated intravascular coagulation (DIC), renal failure, and death. The treatment is supportive.

Inadvertent transfusion of ABO-incompatible blood components resulting in serious harm or death is classified as a Never Event by the Department of Health. All the others are possible consequences of blood transfusion but the symptoms, signs, and timescale support E as the correct answer.

Clevenger B, Kelleher A. Hazards of blood transfusion in adults and children. *Continuing Education in Anaesthesia Critical Care & Pain* 2014; 14 (3): 112–118.

4. E

A trimalleolar fracture cannot be managed conservatively. In general, the second trimester is preferred for semi-elective procedures that can't be deferred until after the baby is delivered. There is no benefit in delaying until the third trimester. Elective surgery should be postponed if possible until at least six weeks post-partum. Lower oesophageal sphincter tone is reduced from early gestation and intra-abdominal pressure increases during the second trimester so an LMA is not recommended. If a general anaesthetic is necessary, it should be a rapid sequence induction

(RSI) with cricoid pressure from the second trimester. Regional anaesthesia is highly desirable as airway management can be more difficult in pregnant patients. The patient would thus maintain her own airway and the spinal would also minimize fetal drug exposure and give good postoperative analgesia. A spinal anaesthetic would therefore be the preferred choice in this patient.

Nejdlova M, Johnson T. Anaesthesia for non-obstetric procedures during pregnancy. *Continuing Education in Anaesthesia Critical Care & Pain* 2012; 12 (4): 203–206.

5. D

Itch is a common side effect of intrathecal opiates. Its mechanism is not fully understood. Opioid itching is not thought to be secondary to histamine release so chlorpheniramine is unlikely to be effective. Prostaglandins are known to modulate c fibre transmission and seem to have a role in opioid induced itch but studies have shown only limited effect form anti-inflammatories like diclofenac. Steroids such as hydrocortisone have no place in the treatment of itch. Opioid antagonists such as naloxone and naltrexone are associated with the greatest success. Low dose is required so as not to reverse the analgesic benefits. Use of ondansetron for pruritis is not first line and evidence for its use is lacking except perhaps in obstetrics.

Hindle A. Intrathecal opioids in the management of acute postoperative pain. *Continuing Education in Anaesthesia Critical Care & Pain* 2008; 8 (3): 81–85.

6. C

The general indications for cell salvage are:
- Surgery where there is expected blood loss >1 L or >20% blood volume, e.g. revision hip replacement
- Preoperative anaemia or major risk factors for bleeding such as Von Willebrand's disease. The WHO classifies anaemia as <13 g/dL in males (<12 g/dL in females)
- Iron deficiency anaemia is common. Normal ferritin levels are 41–400 µg/L
- Patients with rare blood group or antibodies
- Patients who refuse conventional blood transfusion, e.g. Jehovah's Witnesses

Aspirin treatment alone is not a strong indication.

Kuppurao L, Wee M. Perioperative cell salvage, *Continuing Education in Anaesthesia Critical Care & Pain* 2010; 10 (4): 104–108.

7. C

Surgery should be postponed only when there is clear clinical benefit to doing so. Many of the population have an ejection systolic murmur and in the elderly it is often due to aortic sclerosis. Should echocardiography confirm aortic stenosis, there is no reasonable acute treatment to reduce the risk of anaesthesia and hip surgery. Thus there should be no delay awaiting echocardiography. Mild derangement of urea and electrolytes is seen in 40% of patients presenting with a hip fracture. There is commonly a period of dehydration followed by intravenous fluids in hospital. This is not an indication to delay surgery. The patient remains clinically well and respiratory parameters are close to normal for this patient's age with a low oxygen requirement. Atrial fibrillation needs no specific treatment here in the absence of tachycardia. Uncontrolled diabetes with a blood sugar of 16 mmol/L should be controlled acutely prior to surgery. This is well above the normal limit and will become further deranged during surgery. A high glucose will predispose to wound infection. Prosthesis infection is a severe complication when metal is implanted in orthopaedics.

Membership of the Working Party, Griffiths R, Alper J, Beckingsale A, et al. Management of proximal femoral fractures. *Anaesthesia* 2011; 67: 85–98.

8. D

A high-frequency linear probe would provide the best images. A reduced volume of local anaesthetic is likely to be sufficient rather than reduced concentration. The radial nerve will look hyper-echoic. The probe can trace the nerve in the long axis but this block is best performed in the short axis to give a good view of surrounding structures. Use of ultrasound should reduce the risk of intravascular injection but does not remove it and careful aspiration before injection of local anaesthetic is required.

Capek A, Dolan J. Ultrasound-guided peripheral nerve blocks of the upper limb, *Continuing Education in Anaesthesia Critical Care & Pain* 2015; 15 (3): 160–165.

9. A

The cardiovascular compromise is most likely due to the sympathectomy caused by the spinal anaesthetic. Phenelzine is a non-selective irreversible mono-amine oxidase inhibitor. Administration of indirectly acting sympathomimetic agents such as ephedrine or metaraminol may precipitate a severe hypertensive reaction. The next best choice to treat her blood pressure drop secondary to probable vasodilation is phenylephrine. Adrenaline (epinephrine) and noradrenaline (norepinephrine) would be safe to use; however, due to their potency they would not be considered a first line choice.

Bromhead H, Feeney A. Anaesthesia and psychiatric drugs part 1—Antidepressants and anaesthesia. *Anaesthesia Tutorial of the Week* 164. Available at: http://www.frca.co.uk/Documents/164%20 Anaesthesia%20&%20psychiatric%20drugs%20part%201%20-%20antidepressants.pdf

10. D

Blood cultures may be useful to guide antibiotic treatment but can take 48–72 hours to become positive. There is a laboratory result-based risk indicator scoring system for necrotizing fasciitis which gives scores for CRP, WCC, haemoglobin, creatinine level, sodium, and glucose levels. This can help differentiate between cellulitis and necrotizing fasciitis. However, the diagnosis of necrotizing fasciitis is essentially clinical, and D is the gold standard to confirm. Percutaneous needle aspiration may be useful and can be sent for gram stain and culture but tissue biopsy is the investigation of choice. Imaging such as computed tomography or magnetic resonance imaging may be useful but should not delay surgery.

Davoudian P, Flint NJ. Necrotizing fasciitis. *Continuing Education in Anaesthesia Critical Care & Pain* 2012; 12 (5): 245–250.

11. D

This is a question about consent. The operation is urgent rather than emergency so it is reasonable to postpone to allow the patient's wishes to be verified preferably with an advance directive already in place. The family can provide information but ultimately cannot accept nor refuse treatments on behalf of the patient.

AAGBI, Members of the Working Party, Ward ME, Dick J, Greenwell S, et al. *Management of Anaesthesia for Jehovah's Witnesses*, 2nd Edition. AAGBI, 2005, available at: https://www.aagbi.org/sites/default/files/Jehovah's%20Witnesses_0.pdf

12. C

Preoperative anaemia occurs in around 40% of hip fracture patients. It is multifactorial resulting from fracture site bleeding, haemodilution, pre-existing anaemia, or chronic disease. Haemorrhage and haemodilution may result in a fall of around 2.5 g/dL. Anaemic patients are therefore at risk of significant worsening of anaema postoperatively risking ischaemia. Preoperative transfusion should be considered at Hb <9 or Hb <10 for those with a history of ischaemic heart disease as per this case. This patient probably just escapes the need for transfusion preoperatively. If the haemoglobin is 10–12 g/dL, crossmatching 2 units preoperatively and vigilance with respect to intraoperative bleeding should suffice. The surgery planned is not suggested to be more complex and a requirement for a 4-unit transfusion postoperatively would be unusual. Cell salvage is probably more amenable to periprosthetic fracture or revision surgery.

Membership of the Working Party, Griffiths R, Alper J, Beckingsale A, et al. Management of proximal femoral fractures. *Anaesthesia* 2011; 67: 85–98.

13. A

The lateral cutaneous nerve supplies skin sensation over the lateral thigh only. It is a pure sensory nerve. It most often becomes injured by entrapment or compression where it crosses the inguinal ligament near the anterior superior iliac spine peripherally. This is most often seen in association with obesity, but also in other conditions that increase intra-abdominal volume such as pregnancy and ascites, in which the nerve may be kinked or compressed by the bulging abdomen as it leaves the pelvis.

Meralgia paraesthetica is the unpleasant syndrome of paraesthesia and pain in the lateral and anterolateral thigh with no motor weakness. There is no direct thigh injury itself, with the nerve injury being more proximal. This patient's left-sided symptoms are on the non-operative side and may result from a dependent side compression injury during right-sided hip surgery. Usually the condition improves with conservative (non-surgical) treatment. Central damage from complications of neuraxial block is rare.

Khalil N, Nicotra A, Rakowicz W. Treatment for meralgia paraesthetica. *Cochrane Database of Systematic Reviews* 2012; 12: CD004159.

14. D

The number of ribs fractured correlates with the severity of the injury, and together with age they are the most important determinants of morbidity and mortality. Four or more fractured ribs are associated with higher mortality rates and seven or more have a mortality rate of 29%. The associated pain is notoriously difficult to manage, but effective analgesia started promptly prevents hypoventilation, enables deep breathing, adequate coughing with clearance of pulmonary secretions, and compliance with chest physiotherapy. A stepwise multimodal approach to pain should be implemented. This patient is not in a high-risk group and already has reasonable pain control with paracetamol/opioids alone. Additional regional anaesthesia should be considered when pain is not controlled or the patient is at high risk of respiratory complications which often appear 48–72 hours after injury. Potential regional techniques include thoracic epidural, paravertebral, and intercostal blocks or serratus anterior block.

May L, Hillermann C, Patil S. Rib fracture management. *BJA Education* 2016; 16 (1): 26–32.

15. B

Intercostal block carries the highest risk and is a reminder to consider the site of injection as a risk factor for local anaesthetic toxicity. Some sites carry higher risk of direct intravenous injection, e.g. stellate ganglion block, and others carry increased risk of absorption toxicity due to injection into a highly vascular area, e.g. the pleura. In order from lowest to highest risk are subcutaneous, femoral, brachial plexus, epidural, caudal, and intercostal blocks.

Christie LE, Picard J, Weinberg GL. Local anaesthetic systemic toxicity. *Continuing Education in Anaesthesia Critical Care & Pain* 2015; 15 (3): 136–142.

16. D

For this operation profound anaesthesia is required in the distribution of the ulnar and median nerves. If the scar is particularly deep there may be some innervations from the radial nerve from the extensor surface of the hand. Further, a tourniquet will be applied to the upper arm for surgery meaning anaesthesia is required proximal to this level. An axillary block has fewest complications but will commonly miss the intercostobrachial nerve innervating the medial surface of the arm and the lateral cutaneous branches of the radial nerve. An interscalene block is commonly used for shoulder and arm surgery. It does not provide a reliable distal block as commonly misses the inferior trunk and C8, T1 nerve roots. It has a 90% incidence of phrenic nerve palsy on the ipsilateral side and should be avoided in patients with severe respiratory impairment.

A supraclavicular block is a reliable block with fast onset. The three trunks, superior, inferior, and middle, lie close together at this point and are reliably blocked by a single injection. It is performed with the patient in the sitting position and will cover all areas required for arm and hand surgery such that it is referred to as the 'spinal anaesthetic for the arm'. The risk of pneumothorax is minimized by noting the clavicular insertion of sternocleidomastoid muscle. The first rib and dome of the pleura are directly inferior to this point. Keeping the needle insertion point lateral to this landmark in a para-sagittal plane should avoid accidental pleural injury.

New York School of Regional Anaesthesia (NYSORA). Upper extremity blocks. Available at: http://www.nysora.com/techniques/nerve-stimulator-and-surface-based-ra-techniques/upper-extremitya/index.1.html

17. B

All of these techniques may provide analgesia but the adductor canal is the best choice for postoperative analgesia with early mobilization in a day surgery setting. Wound infiltration would be the least effective way of providing good postoperative analgesia. The other blocks are very effective but have more complications including motor block that may affect early mobilization. A femoral nerve block may result in quadriceps weakness and a sciatic nerve block may result in foot drop.

The adductor canal block provides reliable block of the saphenous nerve which is a pure sensory branch of the femoral nerve. The saphenous nerve supplies the medial aspect of the lower leg and foot. This block also blocks the infra-patellar nerve which makes it useful for anterior cruciate repairs and knee arthroscopy procedures. In large volumes, an adductor canal block can provide sensory block of the whole of the front of the knee and can therefore be useful for knee replacements as well.

Quemby D, McEwan A. Ultrasound guided adductor canal (saphenous nerve) block. *Anaesthesia Tutorial of the Week* 301. Available at: https://www.aagbi.org/sites/default/files/301%20Ultrasound%20Guided%20Adductor%20Canal%20(Saphenous%20Nerve)%20Block.pdf

18. C

The over-riding factor is that the patient is in pain and that fractured neck of femur surgery should be expedited to maximize outcome and minimize morbidity associated with bed rest. NICE guideline CG124 updated in March 2014 states operative fixation on the day of admission or the following day reduces the overall mortality risk compared to delayed surgery. There is no objective evidence of correctable arrhythmia at present. Investigations will include 24-hour tape and scanning of carotid arteries. This will add undue delay and be of minimal yield. Surgery should not be further postponed for these reasons.

The history of syncope and blackouts may suggest a cardiac cause so it is pragmatic to avoid spinal anaesthesia in this case as the resulting sympathectomy could have an unpredictable cardiovascular effect. General anaesthesia facilitates easier diagnosis and management of physiological status and emergency treatment if necessary.

There is no indication to withhold beta-blockade when it is an established part of an existing treatment regimen and the heart rate is within normal limits.

NICE Clinical Guideline 124 (2011) Hip fracture management and evidence update. March 2014. Available at: https://www.nice.org.uk/guidance/CG124 https://www.nice.org.uk/guidance/cg124/evidence/evidence-update-183078109

19. D

This clinical picture would fit with bone cement implantation syndrome. This syndrome has no fixed definition but is associated with hypoxia, hypotension, and cardiovascular instability. It tends to occur at the time of cementation, insertion of the prosthesis, reduction of the joint or deflation of the tourniquet. All studies demonstrate right heart failure secondary to increased pulmonary vascular resistance and raised pulmonary artery pressure as the underlying cause. The right ventricle then dilates which reduces the volume of the left ventricle, decreasing its compliance and causing reduced cardiac output.

Khanna G, Cernovsky J. Bone cement and the implications for anaesthesia. *Continuing Education in Anaesthesia Critical Care & Pain* 2012; 12 (4): 213–216.

20. C

Laryngospasm is the sustained closure of the vocal cords resulting in partial or complete loss of the patient's airway. Prompt recognition and early correction is essential to re-establish ventilation and oxygenation.

The patient has signs of laryngospasm, most likely due to painful stimulus and light anaesthesia.

Intravenous propofol will rapidly increase the depth of anaesthesia.

Increasing the sevoflurane to 8% without significantly increasing gas flow will take too long to deepen anaesthesia.

You would increase the FiO_2 to 100% but this will not treat the laryngospasm and be of limited immediate impact in an obstructed airway.

If the above measures fail removal of the LMA or paralysis can be considered.

Gavel G, Walker RWM. Laryngospasm in anaesthesia. *Continuing Education in Anaesthesia Critical Care & Pain* 2014; 14 (2): 47–51.

21. D

Clinically he appears fully reversed; 10 mg of morphine is a relatively small dose for presumably a muscular patient of normal or slightly higher body mass and would not extend so profoundly into the recovery period. Anabolic steroids are more commonly used by body builders who lack concomitant cardiovascular fitness. Professional sportsmen are unlikely to use banned substances. Anxiety would cause a higher respiratory rate with normal or high normal saturations reflecting increased minute volume. Phrenic nerve palsy is a commonly recognized complication of interscalene block, occurring in up to 90% patients. The patient's position should be optimized and he should be monitored in a high-dependency area until the block recedes.

Miller RD, Eriksson LI, Fleisher LA, et al. *Miller's Anesthesia*, 7th Edition. London: Churchill Livingstone 2009, p. 409.

22. E

A femoral nerve block or fascia iliaca block is simple and effective to control preoperative pain. Paracetamol is a good adjunct and is recommended but NSAIDs should be avoided in the elderly population. Entonox provides only temporary analgesia and she has had sufficient opioid that more is unlikely to confer additional significant benefits. Surgery should be planned for the morning.

National Institute for Health and Care Excellence (NICE). *Guidelines. Hip Fracture: The Management of Hip Fracture in Adults*. CG no. 124. London: NICE, 2011.

23. B

Compartment syndrome is a limb threatening condition which causes significant morbidity. Diagnosis is made clinically and a high degree of suspicion is required to ensure prompt intervention. Severe pain that is disproportionate to the degree of injury is the cardinal feature and paraesthesia is characteristic. The most common cause is post fracture in young male patients (<35 years old) and is due to an increase in tissue volume within the compartment. It can occur with open or closed fractures as the skin wound may not decompress the space. Loss of pulses is an uncommon and very late sign. The acute time scale is not consistent with a diagnosis of DVT, cellulitis, or necrotizing fasciitis. There is no erythema on examination, nor signs of systemic sepsis. The acutely ischaemic leg would be cold, white, and pulseless.

Farrow C, Bodenham A, Troxler M. Acute limb compartment syndromes. *Continuing Education in Anaesthesia Critical Care & Pain* 2011; 11 (1): 24–28.

24. B

Atlanto-axial instability can occur in up to 25% of people with rheumatoid arthritis. Anterior subluxation is the commonest and carries the risk of spinal cord compression by the odontoid peg. Anterior subluxation is made worse by neck flexion and therefore can pose significant risks during airway management. Posterior, vertical, and lateral atlanto-axial subluxation are less common as is sub-axial subluxation.

Dislocations are rarer.

Fombon FN, Thompson JP. Anaesthesia for the adult patient with rheumatoid arthritis. *Continuing Education in Anaesthesia Critical Care & Pain* 2006; 6 (6): 235–239.

25. B

The carboxyhaemoglobin level may be up to 15% in heavy smokers. The half-life of carboxyhaemoglobin is 4–6 hours, so overnight abstinence can increase oxygen carriage and delivery which may offer a potential benefit. Also, the haemodynamic effects of cigarette smoke will resolve as nicotine levels return to normal which can take 12–24 hours. Abstinence for over 12 hours can increase physical capacity by 10–20%.

It takes 2–12 days to see an improvement in upper airway reactivity and ciliary function will start to improve after 24 hours as well. It takes two weeks of abstinence to reduce sputum levels to normal levels.

It takes six months to reduce postoperative complication rate to that of the non-smoking population.

Thiagarajan N. Smoking and anaesthesia. *Anaesthesia Tutorial of the Week* 221. Available at: http://www.frca.co.uk/Documents/221%20Smoking%20and%20Anaesthesia.pdf

1. You attend a cardiac arrest call to a medical ward. You arrive to find ward staff administering basic life support to an elderly gentleman with a tracheostomy in situ. Cardiac arrest is confirmed. You are unable to ventilate via the mouth or via tracheostomy. You cannot pass a suction catheter via the tracheostomy. Your next action is:
   A. Attempt oral intubation
   B. Insert laryngeal mask
   C. Remove tracheostomy
   D. Place oxygen over both mouth and tracheostomy
   E. Attempt stoma intubation

2. A healthy volunteer is breathing 80% oxygen for 10 min at sea level. What is the best estimation of partial pressure of oxygen in their alveoli assuming normal diet?
   A. 90 kPa
   B. 88 kPa
   C. 74 kPa
   D. 70 kPa
   E. 61 kPa

3. Which of the following states produce the greatest rightward shift in the oxyhaemoglobin dissociation curve?
   A. Methaemoglobinaemia
   B. Carbon monoxide poisoning
   C. Hyperthermia
   D. Sickle cell anaemia
   E. Massive blood transfusion

4. You anaesthetize a patient for elective DC cardioversion of atrial fibrillation. Which of the following has the least influence on transthoracic electrical impedance?
   A. Obesity
   B. Emphysema
   C. Paddle position
   D. Repeated shocks
   E. Electrode surface area

5. You anaesthetize a 7-year-old boy for emergency exploration of scrotum. You perform rapid sequence induction with thiopentone and suxamethonium, followed by a single dose of rocuronium. Anaesthesia is maintained with oxygen, air, and sevoflurane. You give 3 mg of morphine at the time of incision. After 30 min the groins appear red and warm and you notice blotches developing on the patient's chest and abdomen. You diagnose an allergic reaction. The most likely cause is:

    A. Suxamethonium
    B. Rocuronium
    C. Morphine
    D. Betadine prep
    E. Latex allergy

6. A 54-year-old man has an out of hospital cardiac arrest. There was no bystander cardiopulmonary resuscitation (CPR) performed. He then had 20 min of CPR as per advanced life support (ALS) guidelines until spontaneous return of circulation. He was intubated and ventilated and has been cooled in the intensive care unit (ICU). Which would provide the most accurate predictor of poor neurological recovery?

    A. Bilateral loss of somatosensory evoked potential responses
    B. Seizure activity on electroencephalogram (EEG)
    C. Fixed pupils at 24 hours
    D. Glasgow Coma Scale E1, M2, V1 at 24 hours
    E. Loss of grey–white differentiation on computed tomography (CT) scan at 48 hours

7. You have been called to the Emergency Department for a standby call. A 7-year-old girl has become acutely unwell after ingesting some peanuts. When she arrives her heart rate is 136 bpm and her blood pressure is 81/32 mmHg. She has a widespread urticarial rash with swelling of her lips and tongue. You put 15 L of O_2 on via a trauma mask and call for help. The best immediate action is:

    A. Cannulate and give a 10 mL/kg crystalloid bolus
    B. Intubate with a size 5 endotracheal tube
    C. Give intramuscular adrenaline (epinephrine) 10 µg/kg bolus
    D. Cannulate and give hydrocortisone 100 mg
    E. Secure intra-osseous access and give a 1 µg/kg bolus adrenaline (epinephrine)

8. **A 40-year-old man is brought into the Emergency Department in pulseless electrical activity (PEA) arrest. He was found on the pavement after a night out. There is no evidence of major injury. CPR was commenced immediately and has been on-going for 15 min. He is now intubated and ventilated and his core temperature is 28°C. Which is the most appropriate statement regarding his ongoing resuscitation management?**

   A. Passive warming should be sufficient in raising his temperature
   B. Active external rewarming is sufficient
   C. Fluid restriction is necessary during rewarming
   D. Adrenaline (epinephrine) should be withheld until his temperature is 30°C
   E. Adult life support algorithms should be followed regardless of temperature

9. **A 64-year-old patient complains of central chest pain and nausea. He had a right hemicolectomy two days ago. The pain resolves with oxygen and sublingual glyceryl trinitrate (GTN) spray. His electrocardiogram (ECG) shows flipped T waves in leads V2–V6. His troponin T level 12 hours later is 0.9 mmol/L. His past medical history includes asthma. Which of the following would be the best pharmacological agent to reduce myocardial oxygen demand?**

   A. Propanolol
   B. Aspirin
   C. Diltiazem
   D. Nifedipine
   E. Atenolol

10. **A 26-year-old man has been injured in an explosion. You are the doctor with the pre hospital retrieval team who attends. On examination the patient has suffered traumatic amputation of his right leg above the knee. He is alert and talking and you provide oxygen 100% using a trauma mask. What is the next priority in managing his circulation?**

   A. Cannulate and give 20 mL/kg crystalloid bolus
   B. Cannulate and take blood for haemoglobin estimation and cross match
   C. Apply a tourniquet to his thigh
   D. Apply a pressure dressing to the stump
   E. Cannulate and transfuse O negative blood

11. **A 29-year-old lady presents to the Emergency Department following a sudden collapse at home. She has an uneventful spontaneous vaginal delivery three weeks ago and has been well since. She has a body mass index of 41 and is a smoker. On examination she has a heart rate of 127 bpm, a blood pressure of 65/39 mmHg and oxygen saturations of 87% on 15 L via a trauma mask. She is too unstable to be moved for scanning. What would be the best investigation to help diagnose a pulmonary thromboembolism (PTE)?**

    A. D-dimer level
    B. Chest X-ray
    C. 12 lead ECG
    D. Bedside echocardiography
    E. Arterial blood gas

12. **A 77-year-old man had a prolonged emergency abdominal aneurysm repair 24 hours ago. He is intubated and ventilated in ICU. You notice his abdomen is tense and distended. Over the last 6 hours his urine output has been 5–15 mL/h and his noradrenaline (norepinephrine) requirements have increased. You check his bloods which show a haemoglobin (Hb) of 101 g/L, white cell count of 10.2 × 10⁹/L, and platelets of 154. His urea is 11.6 mmol/L, creatinine 139 μmol/L, and potassium is 5.1 mmol/L. His temperature is 37.3°C. What is the most likely diagnosis?**

    A. Sepsis
    B. Paralytic ileus
    C. Abdominal compartment syndrome
    D. Pancreatitis
    E. Disseminated intravascular coagulopathy

13. **You are called to the Emergency Department to review a 24-year-old man who has been involved in a road traffic accident. He has sustained a head injury and his current Glasgow Coma Scale (GCS) is 4. His pupils are equal and reactive to light. His C-spine is immobilized in a hard collar and he has a 16G intravenous cannula in his right arm. His observations are HR 90 bpm, mean arterial blood pressure 70 mmHg, RR 20, SaO₂ 100% on 15 L of O₂ via a non-rebreathing mask, temperature 35.5°C. There are no other major injuries apparent. The most appropriate next step in the management of this patient is:**

    A. Transfer to radiology for an urgent CT scan of his head and neck
    B. Administration of 100 mL of Mannitol 10% IV
    C. Give a 500-mL fluid bolus
    D. Intubation and controlled ventilation
    E. Discuss transfer with the local neurosurgical centre

14. **You review a 29-year-old woman with brittle asthma on the medical admissions ward. The medical FY2 is concerned as she is not responding to initial treatment. Which feature is most suggestive of life-threatening asthma?**

    A. Peak expiratory flow of 40% predicted
    B. Respiratory rate of 38
    C. Heart rate of 124 bpm
    D. PaCO$_2$ of 5.2 kPA
    E. Patient unable to complete sentences in one breath

15. **A 69-year-old lady presents with a three-day history of severe vomiting. Her arterial blood gases are as follows on room air. pO$_2$ 13.2 kPa, pCO$_2$ 5.9 kPa, H$^+$ 30, HCO$_3^-$ 37 mEq/L. Her U&E are Na$^+$ 139 mmol/L, K$^+$ 2.9 mmol/L, Cl$^-$ 90 mmol/L, urea 8.0 mmol/L, and creatinine 80 μmol/L. What is the most likely diagnosis to account for this biochemical picture?**

    A. Gastroenteritis
    B. Pyloric stenosis
    C. Diabetic ketoacidosis
    D. Renal failure
    E. Cushing's syndrome

16. **You have performed an axillary block for a 54-year-old man. You have just finished injecting 30 mL of 0.5% Bupivacaine. Immediately afterwards he loses consciousness and cardiac arrest is confirmed. You call for help. What is the next step in your management of this patient?**

    A. Give an intravenous bolus of intralipid
    B. Commence CPR
    C. Give an intravenous bolus of adrenaline (epinephrine)
    D. Give an intravenous bolus of amiodarone
    E. Administer an asynchronous shock

17. **A 22-year-old man had a major haemorrhage secondary to trauma. After successful surgery and transfusion of blood products he is now stable. He was given 1 g of tranexamic acid as part of the major haemorrhage protocol. Tranexamic acid is effective in this scenario due to which main action?**

    A. Promoting platelet adhesion and aggregation
    B. Activating the intrinsic arm of the coagulation cascade
    C. Activating the extrinsic arm of the coagulation cascade
    D. Inhibiting monocyte, neutrophil, and complement activity
    E. Inhibiting plasmin formation and displacing plasminogen from fibrin surface

18. **A 28-year-old primigravida survives a major obstetric post-partum haemorrhage requiring massive blood transfusion. She is extubated in ITU. She complains of severe headache, nausea, and vomiting. There is an absence of lactation. On examination she remains hypotensive despite euvolaemia and has bilaterally reduced visual fields. The most appropriate treatment is:**
    A. Thyroxine infusion
    B. Hydrocortisone
    C. Low molecular weight heparin
    D. Progesterone
    E. Oxytocin

19. **The therapeutic effect of adrenaline (epinephrine) administration during cardiac arrest is best explained by:**
    A. Causing tachycardia
    B. Causing peripheral vasoconstriction
    C. Stabilizing mast cell degranulation
    D. Causing bronchodilation
    E. Causing smooth muscle relaxation and sphincter tightening

20. **A 26-year-old intravenous drug user has presented to the Emergency Department. They are in PEA cardiac arrest and CPR is ongoing. A DVT was suspected in his left leg. The only other history was of a right ankle fracture two years ago that required surgical fixation. Two attempts at peripheral IV access by a consultant have failed. The next appropriate step to gain access to the circulation for resuscitation is:**
    A. Site a central line in his right internal jugular vein
    B. Get intraosseous access in his distal right tibia
    C. Get intraosseous access in his left humerus
    D. Site a central line in his right femoral vein
    E. Get intraosseous access in his proximal right tibia

21. **You are called to the ward to deal with a cardiac arrest. When you arrive basic life support has been underway for 2 min. You attach the monitor and diagnose ventricular fibrillation. The best action to take next is:**
    A. Give adrenaline (epinephrine)
    B. Continue chest compressions uninterrupted
    C. Deliver a DC shock to the patient
    D. Intubate the patient
    E. Secure IV access

22. **A 40-year-old, 70-kg man presents to the Emergency Department with severe burns covering an estimated 30% body surface area. It occurred 1 hour ago in a house fire. He smells strongly of alcohol and is violently agitated and confused. ABGs show carboxyhaemoglobin (COHb) is 30%. There is no evidence of an inhalational thermal injury. He requires intubation and ventilation. Which of the following is the most appropriate technique for induction of anaesthesia?**

    A. Inhalational induction with sevoflurane in oxygen
    B. Modified rapid sequence induction with morphine, sodium thiopental, and rocuronium
    C. Rapid sequence induction with propofol and remifentanil
    D. Rapid sequence induction with sodium thiopental and succinylcholine
    E. Fibreoptic intubation under local anaesthesia

23. **A nurse has run through an arterial line ready for the transfer of a patient. You notice there are air bubbles in the tubing connecting the arterial line to the transducer. What is the best description of the resultant changes in the measurement system from this error?**

    A. Damping is increased
    B. Resonance is increased
    C. The systolic blood pressure is over estimated
    D. The minimum bandwidth will be reduced
    E. Less phase shift occurs

24. **An 11-year-old boy presents with an open tibia and fibula fracture sustained playing football whilst on holiday. He is expedited for theatre due to concern about neurovascular compromise. His mother reports a previous anaphylactic reaction under anaesthetic during an elective tonsillectomy two years before, for which he spent 24 hours in intensive care. There are no notes available. He has no medic alert bracelet. Which of the following is best avoided as being the potential causative agent of his previous reaction?**

    A. Penicillin
    B. Latex
    C. Morphine
    D. Sevoflurane
    E. Rocuronium

25. **A 64-year-old man requires rapid sequence induction for surgery for small bowel obstruction. You give thiopentone 5 mg/kg and suxamethonium 1.5 mg/kg. Intubation is unsuccessful and there is now blood in the airway. Bag and mask ventilation is difficult and insertion of a laryngeal mask airway does not improve the situation. There is no CO_2 detected, nor is the chest rising. You declare a can't intubate can't ventilate scenario and proceed to front of neck access to the airway. The best technique to use in this situation is:**

A. Needle cricothyroidotomy

B. Percutaneous tracheostomy

C. Definitive surgical tracheostomy by the general surgeon

D. Scalpel–bougie–cuffed tube tracheostomy

E. Tracheostomy using a cuffed tube and Seldinger technique QuickTrach™ or Melker™

1. C

It is unclear from the immediate history whether the patient has had a previous laryngectomy or not. There is a complete airway obstruction on the basis of inability to ventilate via either route. The inability to pass a suction catheter down the tracheostomy implicates it as the immediate candidate for source of obstruction. It is likely the blocked tracheostomy is obstructing the airway and should therefore be removed first, prior to reassessing. Ventilation via LMA or oral/stoma intubation would be complicated by the original tracheostomy remaining in situ. Placing oxygen on a completely obstructed airway will not help. It would be useful to find out as soon as possible whether the patient has had a previous laryngectomy and how mature the tracheostomy site is.

McGrath BA, Bates L, Atkinson D, Moore JA. Multidisciplinary guidelines for the management of tracheostomy and laryngectomy airway emergencies. *Anaesthesia* 2012, 67, 1025–1041.

2. C

The alveolar gas equation can be used to estimate alveolar oxygen. It is commonly stated as $P_AO_2 = P_iO_2 - P_ACO_2/RQ$. Where P_AO_2 = alveolar oxygen tension, P_iO_2 = inspired oxygen tension, P_ACO_2 = alveolar CO_2 tension, RQ = respiratory quotient. Assuming mixed normal diet, RQ is usually estimated at 0.8. $P_AO_2 = 80 - (5/0.8) = 74$ approximately.

West JB. *Pulmonary Pathophysiology: The Essentials*, 7th Edition. Philadelphia: Lippincott Williams & Wilkins 2007.

3. C

The question is asking in what states does oxygen become more available for tissues. Hyperthermia decreases the oxygen affinity of haemoglobin and therefore makes more oxygen available for tissues. Transfused blood has reduced 2,3 diphosphoglycerate and is less able to deliver oxygen to tissues. Carbon monoxide has 300 times greater affinity for haemoglobin than oxygen, shifting the curve to the left. Similarly, Methaemoglobin (with iron in its oxidized form) is unable to bind with oxygen. Sickle cell is a haemoglobinopathy with less ability to deliver oxygen than HbA.

Thomas C, Lumb AB. Physiology of haemoglobin. *Continuing Education in Anaesthesia, Critical Care & Pain* 2012; 12 (5): 251–256.

4. C

Impedance increases with obesity and emphysema. In repeat shocks, impedance reduces slightly (9%). Impedance reduces with increased electrode size although at the expense of current density. Two paddle positions are commonly described: anteroposterior and anterolateral paddle positions are similar with comparable success rates.

Knowles PR, Press C. Anaesthesia for cardioversion. *BJA Education 2017*; 17 (5): 166–171.

5. E

Despite the vogue for latex free environments, surgical gloves continue to be a source of latex as non-latex gloves are subjectively deemed inferior for precision work. Latex allergy typically occurs 20–40 min into the operation due to direct contact with latex in gloved hands or a reaction to latex particles in the air. Allergy to intravenous drugs used in this case would usually present hyper acutely following their injection. Allergy to betadine (iodine) is less common than latex. Late onset skin irritation may be seen more commonly.

Ryder SA, Waldmann C. Anaphylaxis. *Continuing Education in Anaesthesia Critical Care & Pain* 2004; 4 (4): 111–113.

Mills AT, Paul JA, Ford SM. Anaesthesia-related anaphylaxis: Investigation and follow-up. *Continuing Education in Anaesthesia Critical Care & Pain* 2014; 14 (2): 57–62.

6. A

Accurate neurological prognostication after out of hospital cardiac arrest (OOHCA) is difficult. Although somatosensory evoked potentials are not widely available in the UK, they would provide the most accurate predictor of poor neurological recovery. If they are demonstrated to be bilaterally absent.

One to 3 days after arrest there will be a poor neurological outcome with a false positive rate of 0%. An EEG may unmask subclinical seizures and allow their treatment before neurological status can be checked. Certain other EEG characteristics can be associated with a poor outcome—burst suppression or an isoelectric EEG, but again EEG is not always available. Signs such as fixed pupils and a motor score of 1 on the GCS require a prolonged period of at least 72 hours to be reliable. Loss of differentiation between white and grey matter on a CT scan historically has been thought of as a bad prognostic sign but studies have shown it is not a useful indicator of long-term poor neurological outcome at an early stage.

Temple A, Porter R. Predicting neurological outcome and survival after cardiac arrest. *BJA Continuing Education in Anaesthesia Critical Care & Pain* 2012: 12 (6): 283–287.

7. C

Following the APLS algorithm for emergency treatment of anaphylaxis the first steps are to call for help, remove allergen, administer oxygen via a face mask and administer intramuscular adrenaline (epinephrine) even before assessing airway. The other options are all appropriate management but only after these first four steps have been carried out.

Samuels M, Wieteska S. *Advanced Paediatric Life Support Manual*, 6th Edition. Chichester: Wiley 2016, p. 75.

8. D

In these circumstances rewarming would be best achieved by active internal and external warming as this patient does not have a perfusing rhythm. During rearming vasodilatation will occur so patients will require fluid resuscitation rather than fluid restriction. If the patient's temperature is severely hypothermic adrenaline (epinephrine) should be withheld until the patient has been warmed to above 30°C, then double the interval between adrenaline (epinephrine) doses until the temperature is above 35°C. This is because drug metabolism is slowed and potentially toxic concentrations can be reached with any drug given repeatedly.

Resus Council UK. Advanced Life Support, 7th Edition. 2016. Available at: https://www.resus.org.uk/resuscitation-guidelines/adult-advanced-life-support/

9. C

The immediate management goals in NSTEMI are to prevent new thrombus formation and reduce myocardial oxygen demand. Prevention of new thrombus formation is achieved using platelet inhibition (e.g. aspirin and clopidogrel etc.), and anticoagulation with fondaparinux or sc low molecular weight heparin. To reduce myocardial oxygen demand the first-line agent is a beta-blocker unless contra-indicated. Asthma is a contra-indication to beta-blockers so diltiazem should be used but avoid dihydropyridine calcium channel blocker like nifedipine. Also, if there are signs of left ventricular impairment early introduction of an angiotensin-converting enzyme inhibitor should be considered.

Resus Council UK. Advanced Life Support, 7th Edition. 2016. Available at: https://www.resus.org.uk/resuscitation-guidelines/adult-advanced-life-support/

10. C

The European Guidelines on Advanced Management of Bleeding Care in Trauma (2007, 2010, 2013, 2016) recommend prioritizing prevention of further bleeding by application of tourniquet to an open extremity which is bleeding in the pre surgical setting. Pressure point control is inadequate to control bleeding as collateral circulation is quickly observed. Subsequent management will include estimation of haemoglobin and coagulation status and fluid replacement.

The European Guidelines on Advanced Management of Bleeding Care in Trauma (2007, 2010, 2013, 2016), 4th Edition 2016. Available at: https://www.ncbi.nlm.nih.gov/pmc/articles/PMC4828865/

11. D

The radiological investigation of choice with a suspected PTE is computerized tomographic pulmonary angiography (CTPA). However, this patient's signs and symptoms suggest a massive PTE. When a patient is haemodynamically unstable they should not be moved for radiological investigations.

A portable chest X-ray can be done in the emergency department but is often non-specific.

A bedside echocardiogram can assess for right heart strain/ failure which is more specific to the diagnosis of PTE and may demonstrate a central pulmonary embolism. If echocardiographic findings are suggestive of a PTE, with this clinical picture thrombolysis treatment should be considered.

A 12-lead ECG again has insufficient sensitivity. The ECG may demonstrate sinus tachycardia, atrial fibrillation, right ventricular overload, or right axis deviation. The S1Q3T3 sign is non-specific and is present in <20% of patients with a PTE.

Plasma D-dimer level is only useful if there is low/intermediate clinical probability of a PTE and therefore not in this case.

van Beek EJR, Elliot CA, Kiely DG. Diagnosis and initial treatment of patients with suspected pulmonary thromboembolism. *Continuing Education in Anaesthesia Critical Care & Pain* 2009 (4): 119–124.

12. C

This scenario describes abdominal compartment syndrome which could be secondary to bowel oedema, massive fluid resuscitation, or intra-abdominal bleeding. It should be considered when there is renal, cardiovascular, and respiratory instability. It can be treated with fluids and vasopressors but may require abdominal decompression.

Berry N, Fletcher S. Abdominal compartment syndrome. *Continuing Education in Anaesthesia Critical Care & Pain* 2012; 12 (3): 110–117.

13. D

The patient has an isolated head injury and a low GCS. Therefore the first consideration is airway protection and he requires immediate intubation and ventilation. Optimizing oxygenation and controlling CO_2 will minimize secondary brain injury. Subsequent transfer for imaging will be appropriate when the patient is stable. Discussion with the receiving neurosurgical team will be required to discuss whether operative intervention or specialist management on neuro-intensive care is required. There is no evidence of acutely raised intracranial pressure and no current indication for mannitol to be given. Care should be taken not to fluid overload head injured patients due to the risk of cerebral oedema and secondary hypoxic brain injury. Instead, cerebral perfusion pressure is usually maintained with early use of vasopressors.

Dinsmore J. Traumatic brain injury: an evidence-based review of management. *Continuing Education in Anaesthesia Critical Care & Pain* 2013; 13 (6): 189–195.

NICE: Head Injury: Assessment and Early Management. Clinical Guideline 176, 2014. Available at: Nice.org.uk/guidance/cg176

AAGBI. Recommendations for the Safe Transfer of Patients with Brain Injury. 2006 Available at: www.aagbi.org

14. D

The features of life-threatening asthma are any one of the following:

> Peak expiratory flow (PEF) <33% best or predicted
> SaO_2 <92%
> PaO_2 <8 kPA
> Normal $PaCO_2$ 4.6–6.0 kPa
> Silent chest
> Cyanosis
> Arrhythmia
> Exhaustion
> Altered conscious level
> Hypotension
> Poor respiratory effort

A, B, C, and E are features of acute severe asthma. A normal or rising CO_2 is a feature of life-threatening asthma as it is likely to indicate tiring of respiratory effort and need for intubation and ventilation.

SIGN153. British guideline on the management of asthma, 2016. Available at: https://www.brit-thoracic.org.uk/document-library/clinical-information/asthma/btssign-asthma-guideline-2016/

15. B

This clinical picture of hypokalaemic, hypochloraemic metabolic alkalosis fits with pyloric stenosis. Loss of gastric fluid leads to dehydration and loss of sodium, chloride, acid (H^+), and potassium. The patient requires prompt and adequate fluid and electrolyte resuscitation. In adults this can be secondary to tumours or severe ulcer disease.

Pyloric stenosis: Fluid therapy. *Open Anaesthesia*. Available at: https://www.openanesthesia.org/pyloric_stenosis_fluid_therapy

16. B

The treatment for local anaesthetic toxicity is intralipid but the patient has arrested so the priority is that CPR should be commenced immediately with the intralipid following soon after.

Cave G, Harrop-Griffiths W, Harvey M, et al. AAGBI Local Anaesthetic Toxicity Guidelines 2010. Available at: https://www.aagbi.org/sites/default/files/la_toxicity_2010_0.pdf

17. E

Tranexamic acid inhibits fibrinolysis and promotes clot formation and can reduce bleeding and transfusion requirements. It does also have an anti-inflammatory action.

Reed MR, Woolley T. Uses of tranexamic acid. *Continuing Education in Anaesthesia Critical Care & Pain* 2015; 15 (1): 32–37.

18. B

The patient has features of the rare condition Sheehan's syndrome. This is hypopituitarism caused by ischaemic necrosis due to hypovolemic shock during and after childbirth. It can present as acute failure of anterior pituitary lobe function; the posterior lobe function usually being preserved. Clinical features include severe headache, nausea and vomiting, visual field defects, cranial nerve palsies, and failure of lactation in the parturient. It is treated by management of adrenocortical failure with IV fluids and hydrocortisone replacement.

Kovacs K. Sheehan syndrome. *Lancet* 2003; 361 (9356): 520–522.

19. B

Adrenaline (epinephrine) promotes central circulation to the heart and brain by causing peripheral vasoconstriction. The increased force of vascular contraction improves blood flow to the heart which may help resolve the arrhythmia. All options in this answer correctly describe the range of actions of adrenaline (epinephrine) but only B answers the question by describing which of its effects are being utilized in a cardiac arrest scenario.

Resus Council UK. Advanced Life Support, 7th Edition, 2016. Available at: https://www.resus.org.uk/resuscitation-guidelines/adult-advanced-life-support/

20. C

ALS guidelines recommend intraosseous access where iv access is difficult to establish quickly. It is better to avoid bones that have fractures or orthopaedic pins or plates as this may disrupt the anatomy and circulation. The left humerus is the most appropriate place. Humeral intraosseous placement is associated with higher flow rates and less pain on infusion. This is because, compared to the lower limb bones, it is non-weight bearing and therefore has less bony trabecular mesh in the marrow cavity facilitating ease of infusion. The speed of action of drugs administered via the humerus in comparable to that of an internal jugular central line.

Hoskins SL, Nascimento P Jr, Lima RM, et al. Pharmacokinetics of intraosseous and central venous drug delivery during cardiopulmonary resuscitation. *Resuscitation* 2011; 83 (1): 107–112.

Hoskins SL, Zachariah BS, Copper N, Kramer GC. Comparison of intraosseous proximal humerus and sternal routes for drug delivery during CPR. *Circulation* 2007; 116:II_993.

21. C

The priority in adult ALS is to provide continuous chest compressions, interrupted only to deliver shocks when indicated. The first shock should be given as soon as indicated for in-hospital arrests. Adrenaline (epinephrine) is given every 3–5 min. IV access and intubation can take place at any convenient point in the cycle but should not delay the delivery of shocks. In a pre-hospital scenario it may be reasonable to give 2 minutes of CPR before defibrillation in patients with a prolonged collapse (>5mins).

Resus Council UK. Advanced Life Support, 7th Edition. 2016. Available at: https://www.resus.org.uk/resuscitation-guidelines/adult-advanced-life-support/

22. D

Succinylcholine is safe for the first 24 hours after thermal injury. There is no contraindication to a standard RSI, which is the best technique to intubate the trachea rapidly because a full stomach (alcoholic beverage +/− food) is a distinct possibility and puts the airway at risk from regurgitation/aspiration. Morphine onset/offset is suboptimal for modified RSI.

Bishop S, Maguire S. Anaesthesia and intensive care for major burns. *Continuing Education in Anaesthesia Critical Care & Pain* 2012; 12 (3): 118–122.

23. A

Increased damping is caused by air bubbles, clots, or kinks in the system. Damping is inversely proportional to the third power of the radius, so a small decrease in tubing diameter results in a large increase in damping. As damping is increased, the system is slower to respond to changes in blood pressure and this delay in transducer output is known as phase shift. In the case of under damping, there will be an overshooting response from the system which leads to an overestimation of the pressure change. The minimum bandwidth is independent of the tubing features and describes the range of frequencies over which the transducer system is accurate in vivo. Resonance of the system varies with the amount of damping.

Wilkinson MB, Outram M. Principles of pressure transducers, resonance, damping and frequency response. *Anaesthesia & Intensive Care Medicine* 2009; 10 (2): 102–105.

24. E

The history suggests the patient suffered anaphylaxis during his tonsillectomy. Muscle relaxants are the most common cause of this, accounting for up to 70% of such reactions. Rocuronium is associated with histamine release. Antibiotics are not routinely given for elective tonsillectomy cases. Further precautions are easy to make: using a latex free environment and drugs with lower histamine releasing potential can be substituted (e.g. fentanyl instead of morphine). Sevoflurane is not known to release histamine nor precipitate anaphylaxis.

Harper NJN, Dixon T, Dugué P, Edgar, et al. and Executive Officers, AAGBI (2009), Suspected anaphylactic reactions associated with anaesthesia. *Anaesthesia* 2009; 64: 199–211.

25. D

A scalpel–bougie technique is now the technique recommended by the Difficult Airway Society. It provides a fast and simple technique requiring only basic equipment, readily available where anaesthesia is taking place. A further advantage is that insertion of a cuffed tube provides a degree of security to the airway, allows unobstructed exhalation and monitoring of expired gases including CO_2. Findings of the National Audit Project 4 (NAP4) showed needle cricothyroidotomy to be unreliable in accessing the tracheal lumen and is no longer recommended. Percutaneous tracheostomy is an elective procedure to be carried out in controlled circumstances and a definitive tracheostomy is unlikely to be within the skill set of the surgeons present. Tracheostomy using the Seldinger technique *may* still be used, depending upon the skills and experience of the anaesthetist.

Difficult Airway Society (DAS). Difficult Intubation Guidelines. 2015. Available at: www.dasuk.com

Pracy JP, Brennan L, Cook TM, et al. Surgical intervention during a Can't intubate Can't Oxygenate (CICO) Eve,nt: Emergency Front-of-neck Airway (FONA)?, *BJA: British Journal of Anaesthesia* 2016: 117 (4): 426–428.

4th National Audit Project 2011. Major Complications of Airway Management in the UK. Available at: http://www.rcoa.ac.uk/nap4

1. **A 79-year-old man attends for preoperative assessment prior to bilateral cataract surgery under general anaesthetic. His past medical history includes NYHA grade 3 heart failure. He had an acute coronary event ten months prior for which a drug-eluting stent was placed. He remains on aspirin and ticagrelor. The best management of his thromboprophylaxis in the perioperative period is:**
   A. Stop both antiplatelet agents and proceed
   B. Stop both antiplatelet agents and bridge with IV heparin and proceed
   C. Stop both antiplatelet agents and give platelet transfusion immediately preoperatively
   D. Stop ticagrelor but continue aspirin and proceed
   E. Stop both antiplatelet agents and postpone operation for two months

2. **You perform an awake fibreoptic intubation on a patient with a difficult airway using a spray as you go technique. The maximum described dose for topical administration of lidocaine is:**
   A. 3 mg/kg
   B. 4 mg/kg
   C. 6 mg/kg
   D. 7 mg/kg
   E. 9 mg/kg

3. **You anaesthetize a patient with bowel cancer for elective laparoscopic bowel resection. During laryngoscopy an unanticipated grade 4 larynx is encountered. Mask ventilation and oxygenation are satisfactory. Intubation fails after a total of four attempts at laryngoscopy. The next most appropriate step is:**
   A. Wake the patient, abandon the procedure
   B. Wake the patient, perform awake intubation
   C. Intubate via supraglottic airway device
   D. Scalpel cricothyroidotomy
   E. Maintain oxygenation with nasal high-flow oxygen

4. **You anaesthetize a 17-year-old female for mandibular advancement surgery. The best choice of opioid for cough/gag suppression during extubation is:**

   A. Alfentanil
   B. Fentanyl
   C. Oxycodone
   D. Morphine
   E. Remifentanil

5. **You assess a 23-year-old woman requiring tonsillectomy. She has a history of well-controlled epilepsy and has been seizure free on carbamazepine for three years. Which opioid drug is best avoided in this patient?**

   A. Morphine
   B. Alfentanil
   C. Fentanyl
   D. Diamorphine
   E. Oxycodone

6. **A patient presents for squint surgery. On examination he has one eye where his gaze is deviated laterally and downward. There is an associated unilateral dilated pupil and ptosis. What is the most likely cause?**

   A. Optic nerve palsy
   B. Abducens nerve palsy
   C. Oculomotor nerve palsy
   D. Bell's palsy
   E. Trochlear nerve palsy

7. **A 21-year-old woman with Down's syndrome presents for elective dental extractions under general anaesthesia. Her lead social worker is present. You confirm the patient does not have capacity. Which is the best description of the consent process required?**

   A. The patient can give consent
   B. The patient's next of kin should be sought and asked to give consent on her behalf
   C. The social worker present should give consent on her behalf
   D. An Adults With Incapacity (AWI) form/Consent 4 form should be completed
   E. The anaesthetist and dentist can proceed without consent as acting within the patient's best interest

8. **You anaesthetize a 51-year-old lady for a mastoidectomy. She has well-controlled hypertension and is otherwise well. Her preoperative electrocardiogram (ECG) shows 72 bpm sinus rhythm with a QTc interval of 0.51 seconds. You intend to give her a prophylactic anti-emetic. What would be the best choice for this patient?**

   A. Dexamethasone
   B. Ondansetron
   C. Droperidol
   D. Aprepitant
   E. Metoclopramide

9. **A 48-year-old lady had a total thyroidectomy 3 hours ago. On return to the ward she reports some difficulty breathing and has slowly developed a high-pitched inspiratory noise. On examination, her neck appears more swollen than before. She is haemodynamically stable. You have administered 100% oxygen and called for help. What is the next appropriate management?**

   A. Heliox
   B. Intubate immediately
   C. Nebulized adrenaline (epinephrine)
   D. Remove skin clips
   E. Nebulized steroids

10. **A 68-year-old man is having laser removal of vocal cord tumour. You use a laser endotracheal (ET) tube to secure his airway. What other measure would best minimize the risk of an airway fire?**

    A. Use total intravenous anaesthesia (TIVA) to maintain anaesthesia
    B. Use a nitrous oxide and oxygen mixture
    C. Use the lowest inspired oxygen concentration possible
    D. Put wet swabs around other tissues in the airway
    E. Do not inflate the cuff of the ET tube

11. **A 37-year-old lady had a thyroidectomy for a large multinodular goitre under general anaesthesia with a cervical plexus block for postoperative analgesia. When you review her the next day she is complaining of peri-oral tingling and muscle twitching. Her ECG show a rate of 91 bpm, sinus rhythm with a prolonged QT interval. What is the most likely diagnosis?**

    A. Hypercalcaemia
    B. Hyperkalaemia
    C. Hypomagnesaemia
    D. Hypocalcaemia
    E. Hypokalaemia

12. **A 74-year-old man presents for microlaryngoscopy for suspected tumour. He has a history of alcohol excess and chronic obstructive pulmonary disease (COPD). He reports changes to his voice and dysphagia. Which investigation is best for dynamic airway assessment?**
    A. Magnetic resonance imaging of head and neck
    B. Computed tomography (CT) of head and neck
    C. Flexible nasendoscopy
    D. Chest X-ray
    E. Ultrasound of airway

13. **You have a 74-year-old man for diagnostic laryngoscopy on your ENT list. The surgeon has requested a tubeless field. What is the main advantage of a supraglottic airway approach over a subglottic airway approach be?**
    A. End-tidal CO_2 monitoring is possible
    B. Laser can be used safely
    C. Delivery of a more consistent FiO_2
    D. There is superior access for surgeons
    E. There is a less rapid increase in airway pressures

14. **A 48-year-old lady requires a total thyroidectomy. She is being treated preoperatively with carbimazole and propranolol. What best describes the mechanism of action of propranolol in the treatment of thyrotoxicosis?**
    A. Inhibition of thyroid hormone synthesis
    B. Reduces vascularity of thyroid gland
    C. Reduction in anxiety
    D. Inhibition of peripheral conversion of T4 to active T3
    E. Decreasing amount of thyroid hormone released from the thyroid gland

15. **A patient is admitted to the intensive treatment unit after an uncomplicated neck dissection. His past medical history is otherwise unremarkable. He has a surgical tracheostomy. He has been haemodynamically stable for the past 8 hours since surgery, with oxygen saturation 98% on FiO_2 0.35 with continuous positive airway pressure 5 cmH$_2$O. You are asked to see him as he is gradually desaturating. Currently his SaO$_2$ 91% and he appears anxious and dyspnoeic. You call for help. What is the next most important step?**
    A. Remove the tracheostomy tube and replace with one a size larger
    B. Deliver high-flow 100% oxygen to both face and tracheostomy
    C. Look, listen, and feel at the mouth and tracheostomy
    D. Prepare for oral intubation
    E. Attempt suction of the tracheostomy tube

16. **You anaesthetize a 17-year-old female for surgical extraction of UL8 and LL8 wisdom teeth. She has no significant medical history. The best choice of airway management is:**
    A. Reinforced laryngeal mask
    B. Oral ET tube
    C. Nasal mask
    D. Face mask
    E. Nasal ET tube

17. **A 34-year-old woman presents with goitre requiring elective total thyroidectomy surgery. She has recently been started on inhaled salbutamol for asthma from her GP. Past medical history includes gastritis for which she takes omeprazole. She has been increasingly breathless overnight in bed. She reports difficulty swallowing. Her voice is normal. The most useful investigation preoperatively is:**
    A. Pulmonary function tests
    B. Echocardiography
    C. Flexible nasendoscopy
    D. Upper gastrointestinal endoscopy
    E. CT neck and chest

18. **A 6-year-old child had an elective tonsillectomy which was uncomplicated. The indication was for sleep disordered breathing. Intraoperative analgesia included 2 µg/kg fentanyl, 15 mg/kg paracetamol, and 1 mg/kg diclofenac. In recovery they are distressed and indicate a sore throat. What is the most appropriate initial management?**
    A. Morphine 0.1 mg/kg intravenous bolus
    B. Codeine 1 mg/kg orally
    C. Codeine phosphate 1 mg/kg intramuscularly
    D. Entonox until they calm down
    E. Reassurance from recovery nursing staff

19. **Regarding complications of regional anaesthesia for ophthalmic surgery. The most common complication is:**
    A. Retrobulbar haemorrhage
    B. Globe penetration
    C. Optic nerve injury
    D. Muscle palsy
    E. Chemosis

20. **A 24-year-old man presents with penetrating eye injury requiring urgent surgery. Which anaesthetic induction agent will provide the greatest fall in intraocular pressure?**
    A. Midazolam
    B. Etomidate
    C. Ketamine
    D. Propofol
    E. Thiopental

21. **A 26-year-old woman presents with a five-day history of dental pain due to abscess which the surgeons plan to drain under general anaesthetic. On examination she has mouth opening limited to two finger breadths. Previous anaesthetics as a child were uneventful. She is fasted for more than 6 hours. The best way to anaesthetize this patient is:**
    A. Gas induction
    B. IV induction
    C. Rapid sequence induction
    D. Awake fibreoptic intubation
    E. Ask surgeons to operate under local anaesthetic dental block

22. **A 22-year-old man has sustained a penetrating eye injury as a result of assault. He has been drinking alcohol but is not intoxicated. His Glasgow Coma Scale (GCS) is 15. He has undergone a CT of head which excludes any significant head injury. The ophthalmologist is concerned that any significant delay could jeopardize the sight in this gentleman's eye. What is the most appropriate management plan?**
    A. Perform gas induction with oxygen/nitrous oxide/sevoflurane
    B. Rapid sequence induction (RSI) using thiopentone and suxamethonium 1 mg/kg
    C. Perform an awake fibreoptic intubation
    D. Delay until no longer under the influence of alcohol
    E. Modified RSI with propofol and alfentanil 20 µg/kg

23. **You have a patient on your list for parotidectomy. He is 56 years old and American Society of Anaesthesiologists score (ASA) 1. The surgeon informs you she will be using a facial nerve stimulator. The best technique to facilitate this is:**
    A. Laryngeal mask airway (LMA), spontaneous ventilation
    B. LMA, intermittent positive pressure ventilation (IPPV), without muscle relaxant
    C. Endotracheal tube, IPPV using muscle relaxant at induction only
    D. Endotracheal tube, IPPV without muscle relaxant
    E. ETT, IPPV using suxamethonium at induction only

24. **A 79-year-old female patient with glaucoma presents for cataract surgery under local anaesthesia. The best local anaesthetic to use is:**
    A. Pilocarpine 1%
    B. 2-Chloroprocaine 2%
    C. Lidocaine 2% with 1 in 200,000 adrenaline (epinephrine)
    D. Lidoocaine 2% plain
    E. Levo-bupivicaine 0.5%

25. **You undertake a project examining the time taken in seconds for 30 anaesthetists to perform a fibreoptic intubation on a mannequin. The same anaesthetists then undergo a teaching programme and are timed again. The recorded times indicate an equal mean, mode, and median. The best statistical test to compare the data is:**
    A. t-test
    B. Paired t-test
    C. ANOVA
    D. Paired ANOVA
    E. Wilcoxon signed rank

1. D

Dual antiplatelet therapy is recommended for 12 months following insertion of a drug-eluting stent. During this period, any change to this regimen must balance the risk of bleeding from surgery, the risk of stent occlusion, and the risk of postponing surgery. Stent thrombosis carries a mortality of 45%.

The complex decision making has been simplified into an algorithm shown in Figure 5.1. This allocates patients to a high or low risk of bleeding depending on the type of surgery and then again on the urgency of surgery. In this case the patient is in a low risk situation and answer D is the best answer.

Answer E would also be a reasonable option, accepting that the patient is left awaiting surgery for a further 2 months.

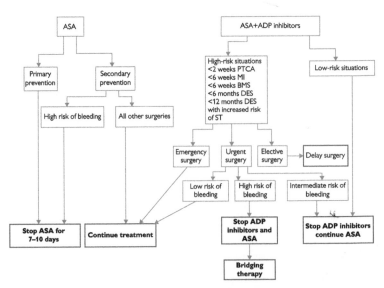

Figure 5.1 Algorithm for perioperative management of antiplatelet therapy ADP, adenosine diphosphate; ASA, aspirin; PTCA, percutaneous transluminal coronary angioplasty; BMS, bare metal stent; DES, drug-eluting stent; MI, myocardial infarction; ST, stent thrombosis

Reprinted from BJA: British Journal of Anaesthesia, 111, A. D. Oprea W. M. Popescu, Perioperative management of antiplatelet therapy pp. i3–i17. Copyright © 2013 The Author(s). Published by Elsevier Ltd. All rights reserved.

Reed-Poysden C, Gupta KJ. Acute coronary syndromes. *BJA Education* 2015; 15 (6): 286–293.

Oprea A, Popescu W. Peri-operative management of anti-platelet therapy. *British Journal of Anaesthesia* 2013; 111: i3–i17.

2. E

Lidocaine is the most widely used agent for topical anaesthesia of the airway using a spray as you go technique. It is available in a variety of strengths and in combination with vasoconstrictors such as adrenaline (epinephrine) and phenylephrine. The maximum described dose for topical administration is 9 mg/kg although doses this high should not be necessary. High doses of local anaesthetics should be used with caution, particularly in patients with liver disease.

Leslie D, Stacey M. Awake intubation. *Continuing Education in Anaesthesia, Critical Care & Pain* 2015; 15 (2); 64–67.

3. C

The question describes an elective case where the patient can be assumed to be fasted. There is no significant history stated regarding reflux. The Difficult Airway Society (DAS) guidance states that the next step is to insert a supraglottic airway device and this can be used as a conduit for intubation. Use of a video laryngoscope should be included during the maximum of four attempts at laryngoscopy. Further attempts should be avoided due to risk of worsening airway trauma and oedema. Clearly there is an emphasis to maintain oxygenation at all times which is being delivered adequately in this case as described.

Frerk C, Mitchell VS, McNarry AF, et al. Difficult Airway Society 2015 guidelines for management of unanticipated difficult intubation in adults. *British Journal of Anaesthesia* 2015; 115 (6): 827–848.

4. E

In certain groups of patients (e.g., neurosurgical, maxillofacial, plastics, and those with significant cardiac or cerebrovascular disease), coughing, gagging, or straining on the ET tube is highly undesirable. The cough suppressant effects of opioid drugs and their ability to attenuate the cardiovascular changes associated with extubation are well known.

Infusion of the ultrashort-acting opioid remifentanil attenuates these undesirable responses and may be used to provide the beneficial combination of a tube-tolerant patient who is fully awake and obeys commands. It is the opioid of choice due to its highly titratable nature.

Popat M, Mitchell V, David R, et al. Difficult Airway Society Guidelines for the management of tracheal extubation. *Anaesthesia* 2012, 67, 318–340.

5. B

Opioid analgesics all possess some degree of proconvulsant activity and are used to enhance EEG activity during seizure focus localization in epilepsy surgery. However, most opioids have a long history of safe use in patients with epilepsy. An exception to this is alfentanil, a particularly potent enhancer of EEG activity, which should be avoided or used with caution.

Carter EL, Adapa RM. Adult epilepsy and anaesthesia. *BJA Education* 2015; 15 (3): 111–117.

6. C

The optic nerve (CN II) transmits visual information. A complete oculomotor nerve palsy will result in a characteristic *down and out* position in the affected eye because the superior oblique (trochlear nerve IV) and lateral rectus (abducens nerve VI) maintain muscle tone compared with all the other paralysed muscles supplied by the oculomotor nerve. In addition, the oculomotor nerve also supplies the upper eyelid muscle (levator palpebrae superioris) and the muscles responsible for pupil constriction (sphincter pupillae). Bell's palsy is a peripheral nerve lesion which affects the facial nerve with an absence of eye signs. Bell's palsy is a peripheral nerve lesion resulting in weakness to the whole half of the face without forehead sparing. A unilateral facial weakness with forehead sparing is usually from a central lesion such as a stroke.

Craven J. Anatomy of the cranial nerves. *Anaesthesia & Intensive Care Medicine* 2010; 11 (12): 529–534.

7. D

The Mental Capacity Act 2005 (England and Wales) and the Adults With Incapacity (Scotland) Act 2000 state that doctors should assume a patient has capacity to consent to treatment unless proven and documented otherwise. This patient has no such capacity and therefore cannot give informed consent.

No adult can give or withhold consent on behalf of another adult.

While it is ideal to involve her parents in preoperative discussions, this has little bearing on the legal, ethical, and professional aspects of the consent process.

Dental treatment is not an emergency procedure therefore there is no scope for the doctor or dentist to proceed without consent 'acting in the patient's best interest'.

An AWI form should be completed by the most senior doctor present.

Adults with Incapacity (Scotland) Act 2000. Available at: http://www.legislation.gov.uk/asp/2000/4/contents

Mental Capacity Act 2005. Available at: https://www.gov.uk/government/collections/mental-capacity-act-making-decisions

Yentis SM, Hartle AJ, Barker IR, et al. AAGBI: Consent for Anaesthesia 2016. Available at: https://www.aagbi.org/sites/default/files/AAGBI%20Consent%20glossy%202016%20consultation%20draft_0.pdf

8. A

The normal range is 0.35–0.44 seconds. Prolonged QTC interval is associated with ventricular arrhythmias. Dexamethasone is a very effective agent for postoperative nausea and vomiting (PONV) prophylaxis with a relative risk reduction of 25% and does not prolong the QTc interval. Droperidol and ondansetron are associated with QTc interval prolongation and should be avoided in patients who exhibit QTc interval prolongation preoperatively. Metoclopramide is not particularly associated with QTc interval prolongation but is a second line choice for postoperative nausea prophylaxis, especially at the 10-mg dose.

Aprepitant is a very effective PONV prophylactic agent and does not prolong the QTc interval. It is not a first line agent due to its high cost but is licensed for chemotherapy-induced nausea and vomiting.

Pierre S. Nausea and vomiting after surgery. *Continuing Education in Anaesthesia Critical Care & Pain* 2013; 15 (1): 28–32.

9. D

This clinical scenario illustrates the postoperative complications of bleeding and haematoma in the neck, post thyroidectomy, causing stridor and external compression of the airway. The next step should be to remove the skin clips to try to release the pressure on the airway. The patient may well need intubation but this may be difficult and the anatomy distorted by the haematoma if it is not released and this should be performed first.

Nebulized adrenaline (epinephrine) and steroid are more useful in the management of stridor secondary to airway oedema.

Heliox may be useful in some cases of stridor but the immediate need here is the evacuation of a haematoma as indicated by neck swelling. Heliox is a mixture of oxygen and helium. It has a similar viscosity to air but a lower density therefore can increase flow and reduce the work of breathing. It has significant effect in the large airways where flow is turbulent and therefore proportional to gas density. Its main uses are for large airway obstruction, e.g. secondary to tumour or oedema, and medium airway obstruction, e.g. croup.

Amphora S. Anaesthesia for thyroid and parathyroid surgery. BJA Education 2007; 7 (2): 55–58.

10. C

The measures recommended to reduce the risk of airway fires are to use air and oxygen mixtures and use low inspired oxygen concentrations, preferably FiO_2 <25% if possible. Wet swabs around the airway tissues can be useful to prevent burns if a fire occurs and the cuff of the ET tube can be filled with saline ± methylene blue to give warning if it has been perforated by the laser.

Itching AJ. Lasers and surgery. BJA Education Review 2003; 3 (5): 143–146.

11. D

Temporary hypocalcaemia requiring replacement occurs in up to 20% of patients post thyroidectomy. Peri-oral tingling, muscle twitching, and tetanic are symptoms of hypocalcaemia, which may progress to seizures or ventricular arrhythmias if untreated. The other biochemical abnormalities are much less likely and would present differently.

Amphora S. Anaesthesia for thyroid and parathyroid surgery. BJA Education 2007; 7 (2): 55–58.

12. C

All of these tests can provide useful information but the gold standard for dynamic airway assessment is the flexible nasendoscopy. If a recent one cannot be found in the notes, or if symptoms have deteriorated, this can be repeated prior to anaesthesia.

Pearson KL, McGuire BE. Anaesthesia for larynges-tracheal surgery including tubeless field. BJA Education 2017; 17 (7): 242–248.

13. D

The main advantage of a supraglottic airway over a subglottic one is that it gives a completely tubeless field and superior surgical access. Supraglottic airway devices do not allow end tidal CO_2 monitoring or delivery of a consistent FiO_2. They also have a more rapid increase in airway pressures with subsequent risk of barotrauma.

Conlon CE. High frequency jet ventilation. Anaesthesia Tutorial of the Week 271. 2012. Available at: https://www.aagbi.org/sites/default/files/271%20High%20frequency%20Jet%20Ventilation[1].pdf

14. D

It is important that the patient is euthyroid before surgery.

Propanolol inhibits the peripheral conversion of T4 to T3 and controls the sympathetic effects of hyperthyroidism.

Other antithyroid drugs include: carbimazole, which prevents thyroid hormone synthesis; propylthiouracil, which inhibits conversion of T4–T3; iodine (Lugol's solution), which inhibits thyroid hormone production and reduces the vascularity of the thyroid gland.

Davis S, Adams L. Anaesthesia for thyroid surgery. *Anaesthesia Tutorial of the Week* 162. 2009. Available at: http://www.frca.co.uk/Documents/162%20Anaesthesia%20for%20thyroid%20surgery.pdf

15. C

After calling for help, you must next look, listen, and feel for breathing at both the mouth and tracheostomy. This may be aided by waveform capnography if available, or use of a Mapleson C breathing system and reservoir bag. This ascertains the presence or absence of a patent airway at both sites and whether spontaneous breathing is present.

When breathing is present, oxygen should be applied to both mouth and tracheostomy. If breathing is absent then a pulse check ± CPR is carried out.

Attempting suction of the tracheostomy tube may potentially dislodge any obstructing clot or mucus further down the respiratory tract. Removing the tube from an acutely formed tracheostomy will lead to loss of the tract and potentially the whole airway.

McGrath BA, Bates L, Atkinson D, Moore JA. Multidisciplinary guidelines for the management of tracheostomy and laryngectomy airway emergencies. *Anaesthesia* 2012; 67: 1025–1041.

16. B

The airway should be protected from blood and dental foreign bodies by a cuffed ET tube. A nasal tube is best indicated to facilitate surgical access when the dental extractions are bilateral. However, on this occasion both wisdom teeth are on the left side (upper left and lower left) so an oral ET tube can be placed and manoeuvred to the opposite side. This prevents the risk of nasal trauma from a nasal tube yet still facilitates unilateral surgical access.

Cantlay K, Williamson S, Hawkings J. Anaesthesia for dentistry. *Continuing Education in Anaesthesia Critical Care & Pain* 2005; 5 (3): 71–75.

17. E

A large retrosternal goitre causing tracheal compression symptoms in the mediastinum when lying flat should be excluded. The patient is at risk of tracheomalacia. Further enlargement may also result in dysphagia and recurrent laryngeal nerve palsy. Chest X-ray may show tracheal impression but CT scan is the gold standard and will give more detailed information. Severe heart failure and adult-onset asthma are worth investigating after identifying an absence of thyroid compressive causes. Pulmonary function tests are likely to show obstruction in both asthma and external compression so may not narrow the differential diagnoses. There are no obvious features of severe reflux and the patient is already on proton pump inhibitor therapy.

Malhotra S, Sodhi V. Anaesthesia for thyroid and parathyroid surgery. Continuing Education in Anaesthesia Critical Care & Pain 2007; 7 (2): 55–58.

18. A

The history of sleep-disordered breathing implies obstructive sleep apnoea, an indication for tonsillectomy. A 6-year-old child should be deemed able to reliably communicate and indicate pain. Simple reassurance alone is therefore inadequate. Codeine is contraindicated due to genetically determined variations in metabolism (different CYP 2D6 phenotypes including ultrarapid metabolizers who are at risk of toxicity, and slow metabolizers in whom codeine has an inadequate effect due to lack of metabolism to morphine, its active form). The child is sore and requires strong analgesia. The pain is likely to persist in the medium term so entonox is not optimal. A strong opioid such as morphine is indicated and has a more predictable dose response. The dose is correct being 0.1–0.2 mg/kg IV.

Hansen J, Shah R, Benzon H. Management of pediatric tonsillectomy pain: A review of the literature. *Dovepress* 2016; 3: 23–26.

Ravi R, Howell T. Anaesthesia for paediatric ear, nose, and throat surgery. *Continuing Education in Anaesthesia Critical Care & Pain* 2007; 7 (2):, 33–37.

Williams DG, Patel A, Howard RF. Pharmacogenetics of codeine metabolism in an urban population of children and its implications for analgesic reliability. *British Journal of Anaesthesia* 2002; 89 (6): 839–845.

19. E

Chemosis is a swollen conjunctiva which subsides with compression and the passage of time. All the others are much rarer complications. There have been no large randomized studies to compare risks of complications between methods of local anaesthesia. Selection of technique therefore remains largely a matter of personal preference and expertise.

Parness G, Underhill S. Regional anaesthesia for intraocular surgery. *Continuing Education in Anaesthesia Critical Care & Pain* 2005; 5 (3): 93–97.

20. D

All IV induction agents lower IOP except ketamine. Thiopental, propofol, and etomidate all cause a fall in IOP. The fall is greatest with propofol, but at the cost of a greater reduction in arterial pressure. Induction agents which cause myoclonus, such as etomidate, should not be given in perforating eye injuries. Midazolam has no effect on IOP.

Raw D, Mostafa SM. Drugs and the eye. *BJA CEPD Reviews* 2001; 1 (6): 161–165.

21. D

The airway is made difficult by the reduced mouth opening. The only method which avoids this problem is awake fibreoptic nasal intubation. After five days this restriction is unlikely to improve pre-induction with analgesia and will perhaps improve only slightly after a gas induction. Access via the mouth will remain problematic. This together with the abscess will preclude effective local anaesthetic.

Difficult Airway Society. Awake fibre optic intubation. Available at: https://www.das.uk.com/content/patient_info/what_is_awake_fibre_optic_intubation

Leslie D, Stacey M. Awake intubation. *Continuing Education in Anaesthesia Critical Care & Pain* 2015; 15 (2): 64–67.

22. B

D is inappropriate given not clinically intoxicated and negative CT head.

A is inappropriate due to potentially full stomach and increase in intra-ocular pressure due to nitrous oxide.

C is inappropriate due to interaction of alcohol and sedative drugs. Without sedation hypertension is likely which may cause an increase in IOP.

E is still a full stomach scenario therefore a muscle relaxant for optimal intubating conditions should be used.

Anaesthesia UK. Anaesthesia for miscellaneous surgery. Available at: http://www.frca.co.uk/article.aspx?articleid=100700

Wilson A. Anaesthesia for Emergency eye surgery. *Update in Anaesthesia.* Available at: http://e-safe-anaesthesia.org/e_library/06/Anaesthesia_for_emergency_eye_surgery_Update_2000.pdf

23. D

The surgeon's use of a facial nerve stimulator requires the neuromuscular junction to be intact and functioning normally. Non-depolarizing muscle relaxants should be avoided as these will lead to false negatives on facial nerve testing. Suxamethonium could be used at induction but this assumes the patient is of normal phenotype to ensure the block is not unduly prolonged. An LMA technique is not recommended for this operation as the surgeon requires to move the head, and venous pressure and pCO_2 must be controlled.

Remifentanil can be used from induction through maintenance to ensure balanced anaesthesia deep enough to permit ventilation without excessive volatile agent concentrations or muscle relaxant.

Allman K, Wilson I, O'Donnell A. Anaesthesia for ENT surgery. In *Oxford Handbook of Anaesthesia*, 4th Edition. Oxford: Oxford University Press, 2016; Chapter 26.

24. D

Lidocaine 2% plain is a safe, short acting amide local anaesthetic with fast onset making it ideal for cataract surgery. There is little post operative pain so longer acting drugs such as levo-bupivicaine have no additional benefit.

Adrenaline (epinephrine) is a sympathomimetic and has a vasoconstricting effect. Adrenaline (epinephrine) containing solutions often contain preservative sodium metabisulphite also, which is potentially toxic to the globe. Adrenaline (epinephrine) can be absorbed systemically producing tachycardia, arrhythmias, and hypertension. As such, these solutions are avoided.

Pilocarpine is a parasympathomimetic agent used when miosis is required and has no local anaesthetic activity.

2-Chloroprocaine is a newer ester type local anaesthetic most commonly used in the USA at present.

e-learning for health. Local anaesthesia pharmacology for ophthalmic surgery. Available at: http://portal.e-lfh.org.uk/LearningContent/Launch/450909

25. B

The data collected are quantitative not qualitative. The equal mean, mode, and median indicate a normal distribution. There are two groups made up of the same sample repeated, therefore a paired t-test is most appropriate to examine for significant difference between the groups. ANOVA is more appropriate for more than two normally distributed groups. Wilcoxon is more appropriate for non-normally distributed (skewed) data.

Kestin I. Statistics in medicine. *Anaesthesia and Intensive Care Medicine* 2012; 13(4): 181–188.

1. **You anaesthetize a patient for laparoscopic nephrectomy which has now been converted to an open procedure. You recommend that the patient should receive a continuous local anaesthetic wound infiltration catheter. The surgeon asks where is best to place it?**
   A. Subcutaneously
   B. Between external oblique and internal oblique muscle layers
   C. Between internal oblique and transversus abdominis muscle layers
   D. Preperitoneal
   E. Intraperitoneal

2. **Regarding patient positioning under general anaesthesia. The most commonly reported nerve injury postoperatively is:**
   A. Ulnar nerve
   B. Common peroneal nerve
   C. Lateral cutaneous nerve of thigh
   D. Median nerve
   E. Sciatic nerve

3. **You anaesthetize a 71-year-old woman for day surgery laparoscopy. She has a history of early Parkinson's disease which is well controlled. Her drug therapy includes ropinirole. The best choice of antiemetic is:**
   A. Prochlorperazine
   B. Metoclopramide
   C. Droperidol
   D. Ondansetron
   E. Domperidone

4. **You anaesthetize a 66-year-old man for open cholecystectomy. He has moderate chronic obstructive pulmonary disease (COPD). His current ventilation settings are FiO$_2$ of 0.5, P insp of 25 cmH$_2$O, PEEP 6 cmH$_2$O, I:E ratio of 1:2 with a RR 12 bpm giving a tidal volume of around 500 mL. You notice his blood pressure has dropped to 90/42 and his tidal volume has dropped to 390 mL. The expiratory flow does not return to zero prior to inspiration. He is adequately paralysed. What is the best ventilatory management at this point?**

    A. Switch to volume controlled ventilation
    B. Increase the I:E ratio to 1:4
    C. Increase the P insp to 30 cmH$_2$O
    D. Decrease the respiratory rate to 8
    E. Decrease the PEEP to 0

5. **An ASA1 42-year-old-female patient had an uneventful laparoscopic cholecystectomy. In recovery she develops inspiratory stridor and tachypnoea and has desaturated to 90% on 6 L of oxygen via a Hudson mask. You have called for help and performed a jaw thrust with no improvement. What is the next most appropriate management?**

    A. Give propofol
    B. Give suxamethonium
    C. Give nebulized salbutamol
    D. Application of CPAP with 100% oxygen with Mapleson C system
    E. Perform a rapid sequence induction and re-intubate

6. **A 54-year-old lady in the HDU is receiving an amiodarone infusion for fast atrial fibrillation. You review her 3 hours later because she is complaining of pain in her arm around the cannula site where the amiodarone is being infused. You note the area is swollen, tense, and red. You immediately stop the infusion and aspirate as much as you can from the cannula and elevated her arm. What is the most useful secondary management to reduce tissue injury?**

    A. Stellate ganglion block
    B. Intravenous hydrocortisone
    C. Saline washout
    D. Phentolamine injection
    E. Hyaluronidase injection

7. **A 58-year-old male presents for carotid endarterectomy (CEA) after an episode of amaurosis fugax in the right eye. He has been commenced on clopidogrel. He is awaiting three vessel coronary artery bypass graft (CABG) for angina which is stable. He also has hypertension and hypercholesterolaemia. His other medications are aspirin, amlodipine, ramipril, simvastatin, isosorbide mononitrate, nicorandil, and glyceryl trinitrate (GTN) spray as required. What is the single most appropriate action plan?**

   A. Cancel CEA until CABG, continue clopidogrel
   B. Proceed with right CEA and continue clopidogrel
   C. Cancel CEA and proceed with CABG but stop clopidogrel
   D. Proceed with left CEA and stop clopidogrel
   E. Proceed with right CEA and stop clopidogrel

8. **Regarding monitoring of non-depolarizing neuromuscular blockade, which statement is the most accurate?**

   A. A train of four >0.8 is a reliable indicator of return of safe motor function
   B. Should commence pre-induction and continue until a reversal agent is given
   C. Can be done using the isolated forearm procedure
   D. Total paralysis is evidenced by continued apnoea
   E. Is accurate using a quantitative monitor of measurement

9. **A 26-year-old female presents with neuropathic pain and paraesthesia along the lateral border of her hand for six months. On examination she has wasting of the abductor pollicis brevis, the hypothenar eminence, and the interossei muscles of the hand. There is no history of trauma. The most likely diagnosis is:**

   A. Radial nerve palsy
   B. Carpal tunnel syndrome
   C. Thoracic outlet syndrome affecting C8 and T1 nerve roots
   D. Raynaud's disease
   E. Median nerve palsy

10. **A 62-year-old man with COPD and hypertension is recovering from a laparotomy for a perforated duodenal ulcer. He can now eat and drink and is to convert from his patient-controlled anaesthesia morphine to oral analgesia. He has used 40 mg IV morphine in the last 24 hours. What would be the most appropriate oral analgesia regimen?**

    A. Six hourly co-codamol 30/500
    B. Six hourly tramadol 100 mg
    C. MST 40 mg bd with 10 mg sevredol for breakthrough and regular paracetamol
    D. MST 20 mg bd with 5 mg sevredol for breakthrough and regular paracetamol
    E. Regular co-codamol 30/500 mg with tramadol 100 mg for breakthrough

11. **A 34-year-old female with myotonic dystrophy requires a laparoscopic cholecystectomy. She has a body mass index (BMI) of 38. She has a normal airway and no symptoms of reflux. She has had her usual medications. The surgeon requests muscle relaxation for the operation. What would be the best option for muscle relaxation?**

    A. Use a reduced dose of rocuronium with sugammadex for reversal

    B. Use an increased dose of rocuronium with sugammadex for reversal

    C. Use usual dose of suxamethonium with no reversal agent

    D. Use a reduced dose of rocuronium with glycopyrrolate/neostigmine for reversal

    E. Use an increased dose of vecuronium with glycopyrrolate/neostigmine for reversal

12. **You anaesthetize a 71-year-old man for elective abdominal aortic aneurysm repair. He is stable following epidural insertion and induction of anaesthesia. The surgeon tells you he is about to cross clamp the aorta. What is the next step in your anaesthetic management of this patient?**

    A. Administer a bolus of local anaesthetic epidurally

    B. Have a noradrenaline (norepinephrine) infusion ready for immediate use

    C. Start volume loading the patient

    D. Deepen anaesthesia

    E. Increase the FiO_2 to 1.0

13. **A 72-year-old man requires an emergency laparotomy. A CT scan has shown a perforated diverticulum. He has a past medical history of atrial fibrillation and hypertension. His heart rate is AF 110, blood pressure 97/63, and temperature 38.5°C. The surgeons are keen to proceed. The most appropriate risk assessment tool is:**

    A. ASA grade

    B. Lee's RCRI

    C. P-POSSUM score

    D. HES procedure group

    E. APACHE-II score

14. **A 72-year-old female patient with chronic renal failure has notoriously difficult peripheral and central IV access. She had multiple central lines over the last 20 years. She requires an upper body central line. The *gold standard* test to check catheter tip position is:**

    A. Chest X-ray

    B. Ultrasound/echocardiography

    C. Arterial blood gas analysis

    D. Fluoroscopy with contrast

    E. Monitored pulse waveform

15. **A 77-year-old man is recovering well after an anterior resection. His epidural catheter has been removed after providing successful analgesia for 72 hours. He has chronic atrial fibrillation and is on rivaroxaban. What is the safe minimum time interval to recommence his rivaroxaban after the epidural catheter has been removed?**

    A. 1 hour
    B. 6 hours
    C. 12 hours
    D. 24 hours
    E. 48 hours

16. **A 35-year-old female patient is undergoing elective laparoscopic cholecystectomy. She is ASA grade 1 and describes significant reflux symptoms. She has an uneventful rapid sequence induction of anaesthesia and is maintained on oxygen/air/volatile agent. During surgery she becomes significantly tachycardic, hypercapnic with increasing oxygen requirements, and increasing muscle tone. Her temperature is 39.9°C. The most immediate clinical priority is:**

    A. Dantrolene 2.5 mg/kg immediate IV bolus
    B. Change to volatile free anaesthetic machine
    C. Calcium chloride 10% 10 mL IV bolus
    D. Magnesium sulphate 8 mmol slow IV bolus
    E. Begin active cooling

17. **A 38-year-old man presents vomiting copious fresh red blood. He has a history of alcohol excess. He is responding to resuscitation measures and requires urgent upper gastrointestinal endoscopy. He is commenced on IV omeprazole. What additional drug is most useful?**

    A. Somatostatin
    B. Octreotide
    C. Erythromycin
    D. Vasopressin
    E. Terlipressin

18. **You are competently preoxygenating a patient for rapid sequence induction of anaesthesia. The best indicator of adequate preoxygenation is:**

    A. Presence of full capnograph trace with respiration
    B. Absence of gas leak around tight fitting face mask
    C. Reservoir bag movement with respiration
    D. End tidal oxygen fraction ≥0.9
    E. Timed ≥3 min of preoxygenation

19. **A sample of 100 patients, suspected of having a disease, undergo a test. Eighty of the patients test positive for the disease. In reality, only 60 of these patients actually have the disease. What is the positive predictive value of the test?**

    A. 25%

    B. 40%

    C. 60%

    D. 75%

    E. 80%

20. **An unfasted patient with known homozygous serum cholinesterase deficiency and severe gastro-oesophageal reflux undergoes emergency laparoscopic appendicectomy. A modified rapid sequence induction is performed using rocuronium 1.0 mg/kg and his trachea is intubated without difficulty. At the end of surgery, the rocuronium is reversed with sugammadex. However, only 2 hours later it is necessary to return the patient to theatre for control of brisk bleeding. The patient has already eaten a meal. Which of the following muscle relaxants is it safest to use?**

    A. Atracurium

    B. Mivacurium

    C. Rocuronium

    D. Succinylcholine

    E. Vecuronium

21. **A 56-year-old woman who has a BMI 55 kg/m² remains in the recovery room following an uneventful but prolonged laparoscopic cholecystectomy. It finished over an hour ago. Her oxygen saturation is 85% on room air but rises to 99% when 2 L/min oxygen is delivered via nasal prongs. All other observations are within normal limits. The most likely cause of her ongoing hypoxaemia is:**

    A. Hypoventilation

    B. Atelectasis

    C. Pulmonary micro-embolism

    D. Diffusion hypoxia due to nitrous oxide

    E. Residual neuromuscular blockade

22. **A 53-year-old woman is in recovery following elective laparoscopic resection of unilateral phaeochromocytoma. She is complaining of light-headedness. Her blood pressure is 71/29 with heart rate of 74. Surgery was otherwise uneventful. Her fluid balance appears appropriate and there is no sign of bleeding. Preoperatively she was stable on phenoxybenzamine and atenolol. The most appropriate initial drug therapy is:**
    A. Vasopressin
    B. Enoximone
    C. Dobutamine
    D. Noradrenaline (norepinephrine)
    E. Adrenaline (epinephrine)

23. **You anaesthetize a patient for open abdominal aortic aneurysm repair. The graft is now complete and the surgeon has released the aortic cross clamp resulting in a sudden drop in blood pressure to 65/35. The mechanism of hypotension is primarily caused by:**
    A. Ischaemia–reperfusion injury
    B. Lactic acidosis
    C. Decreased coronary blood flow
    D. Blood sequestration in the lower half
    E. Reduced peripheral vascular resistance

24. **You anaesthetize a patient for repair of ruptured abdominal aortic aneurysm. He was cardiovascularly unstable requiring resuscitation preoperatively. Suprarenal cross clamp of the aorta was used briefly. The best way to avoid postoperative renal dysfunction is:**
    A. Ensure adequate extracellular fluid volume
    B. Give mannitol intraoperatively
    C. Give furosemide intraoperatively
    D. Give dopamine intraoperatively
    E. Give bicarbonate loading dose intraoperatively

25. **You have a patient present for an elective mastectomy with a history of severe postoperative nausea and vomiting. You decide to manage this patient with TIVA (total intravenous anaesthesia) using target-controlled infusions (TCIs) of propofol and remifentanil. Which of the following statements best describes TCI propofol?**
    A. The Minto model is the most commonly used
    B. The k_{eo} value in the Schnider model refers to the plasma concentration
    C. The Schnider model will give a more accurate wake up time compared to the Marsh model for obese patients
    D. The Marsh model will make adjustments for advanced age
    E. Propofol TCI is a combination of three different infusions rates operating simultaneously and controlled by a microprocessor

1. C

The innervating nerves run between the muscle layers internal oblique and transversus abdominis, which is the best site for catheter placement, similar to the anatomy of a TAP block. There remains some controversy over the exact placement of wound catheters at various surgical sites. Placing the catheter between muscle layers requires a layered wound closure by the surgeon.

Whiteman A, Bajaj S, Hasan M. Novel techniques of local anaesthetic infiltration. *Continuing Education in Anaesthesia, Critical Care & Pain* 2011; 11 (5): 167–171.

2. A

More than a quarter of all perioperative nerve injuries involve the ulnar nerve. The classic site of injury is in the ulnar groove behind the medial epicondyle of the humerus. At this point, the nerve is quite exposed to both direct trauma from the sides of the operating table and indirect trauma from stretch. It is three times more common in males than females.

Knight DJW, Mahajan RP. Patient positioning in anaesthesia. *Continuing Education in Anaesthesia, Critical Care & Pain* 2004; 4 (5): 160–163.

3. D

Parkinson's disease is a common neurodegenerative disorder due to loss of dopaminergic neurones in the substantia nigra. Ropinirole is a dopamine agonist. A number of anti-emetics are contraindicated in Parkinson's disease due to their dopamine antagonist effects. 5-HT$_3$ receptor antagonists (e.g. ondansetron) and H$_1$-receptor antagonists have fewer side effects.

Chambers DJ, Sebastian J, Ahearn DJ. Parkinson's disease. *BJA Education* 2017; 17 (4): 145–149.

4. B

This clinical scenario suggests 'breath stacking' when airway narrowing limits expiratory flow causing inspiration to occur before expiration is complete. This leads to development of intrinsic PEEP, raised intrathoracic pressure, and potential cardiovascular instability due to decreased venous return.

Allowing more time for expiration either by increasing the I:E ratio or decreasing the respiratory rate would allow more time for exhalation and reduce the likelihood of breath stacking. However, decreasing the respiratory rate too much may cause hypercapnia, acidosis, and hypoxia so a balance needs to be achieved. A respiratory rate of 8 is probably too low.

Increasing the P insp would increase the chance of barotrauma.

Switching to volume-controlled ventilation would cause an increase in peak pressure again with a risk of barotrauma.

Increasing PEEP rather than decreasing it could be beneficial by keeping small airways open during exhalation but again at risk of cardiovascular compromise if too high.

Lumb A, Biercamp C. Chronic obstructive pulmonary disease and anaesthesia. *Continuing Education in Anaesthesia Critical Care & Pain* 2014; 14 (1): 1–5.

5. D

The symptoms of stridor, tachypnoea, and desaturation postoperatively suggest laryngospasm, which requires prompt recognition and treatment. As this patient has no airway device in place the initial step would be to apply CPAP with 100% oxygen and potentially the laryngospasm will resolve. If this fails you may need to progress to treatment with propofol ± suxamethonium and may need to secure the airway with an endotracheal tube.

Gavel G, Walker RWM. Laryngospasm in anaesthesia. *Continuing Education in Anaesthesia Critical Care & Pain* 2014; 14 (2): 47–51.

6. C

Extravasation of amiodarone can lead to tissue necrosis. Saline washout under local or general anaesthesia is probably the most effective treatment to remove and dilute the drug from the site of injury and has been shown to reduce tissue injury.

Steroids have been used historically but there is little evidence to support their use after extravasation injuries.

Hyaluronidase has a temporary effect of making tissues more permeable when injected at the site which could help dispersion of extravasated amiodarone. It could therefore aid a saline washout but is of no benefit alone.

Phentolamine injected at the site can relax smooth muscle and cause vasodilatation. Early use is only recommended after extravasation of vasopressors.

Stellate ganglion block can again cause vasodilatation and may have a role after the extravasation of vasopressors and thiopentone only. The procedure also has risks and side effects to be considered.

Lake C, Beecroft CL. Extravasation injuries and accidental intra-arterial injection. *Continuing Education in Anaesthesia Critical Care & Pain* 2010; 10 (4): 109–113.

7. B

Proceed with right CEA and continue clopidogrel.

In terms of which procedure first, CABG is a major cardiovascular risk procedure. CEA is intermediate. Therefore, performing CEA before CABG is overall the most cardiovascular protective strategy. With the symptom of Amaurosis fugax, the carotid lesion is ipsilateral. A number of studies have shown that stopping antiplatelet therapy prior to CEA increases the risk of stroke while presenting only a moderate bleeding risk.

Ladak N, Thompson J. General or local anaesthesia for carotid endarterectomy? *Continuing Education in Anaesthesia Critical Care & Pain* 2012; 12 (2): 92–96.

8. E

The muscular response to ulnar nerve stimulation is best but the facial or peroneal nerves can also be used. Monitoring of neuromuscular blockade using a peripheral nerve stimulator is essential for all stages of anaesthesia when neuromuscular drugs are administered. It should be commenced at induction to ensure adequate relaxation prior to intubation and continued until return of consciousness.

Awareness is most common at induction and during transfer from the anaesthetic room to theatre (50% cases), and around 20% of cases occur during emergence, commonly related to inadequate reversal of neuromuscular block.

The isolated forearm technique is a monitor of awareness, not neuromuscular block.

Train of four (TOF) monitoring must be quantitative to be accurate. Trials have shown marked inadequacy of qualitative assessment methods, even with experienced anaesthetists.

McGrath CD, Hunter, JM Monitoring of neuromuscular block. *Continuing Education in Anaesthesia Critical Care & Pain* 2006; 6 (1): 7–12.

National Audit Project 5. Accidental Awareness under General Anaesthesia (AAGA). RCoA and AAGBI September 2014. http://www.nationalauditprojects.org.uk/NAP5report

Viby-Mogensen J, Jensen NH, Engbaek J, et al. Tactile and visual evaluation of the response to train-of-four nerve stimulation. *Anesthesiology* 1985; 63: 440–443.

9. C

This description describes neurogenic thoracic outlet syndrome involving C8 and T1 nerve roots with pain, paraesthesia, and muscle wasting in an ulnar distribution. This is the most common neurogenic type although radial nerve symptoms and referred pain to chest, neck, ear, and upper arm from C5, C6, and C7 involvement can also be present sometimes. Thoracic outlet syndrome most commonly affects young females between the ages of 20 and 40 years.

Lewis J, Telford R. Anaesthesia for vascular surgery of the upper limb. *Continuing Education in Anaesthesia Critical Care & Pain* 2014; 14 (3): 119–124.

10. D

This gentleman has had the oral equivalent of 80 mg of morphine in the last 24 hours and is likely to need stronger opioids than just co-codamol and tramadol initially. It is reasonable as a starting measure to prescribe half this dose in a modified release opioid form. Half this should be given in the morning and half in the evening. Extra doses of short-acting opioids must be available regularly for breakthrough.

Conversion of IV to oral morphine is a 1:2 ratio.

BNF. Pain management with opioids. Available at: http://www.evidence.nhs.uk

Pain data pain management opioid conversion calculator. Available at: http://www.paindata.org/calculator.php

11. A

Myotonic dystrophy is an autosomal dominant disorder. Multisystem signs and symptoms usually manifest in early adulthood. They have myotonia which is incomplete muscle relaxation, especially the inability to 'let go' after a hand grip. They may also have muscle wasting, cardiac and respiratory abnormalities, endocrine dysfunction, and intellectual impairment.

Depolarizing neuromuscular blocking agents and anticholinesterase drugs may induce generalized muscle contractures and should be avoided.

Non-depolarizing neuromuscular blocking agents are not associated with myotonia but patients with this disease may show increased sensitivity to them. If they are absolutely required, they should be given in reduced doses with careful monitoring and sugammadex to ensure complete reversal.

Marsh S, Pittard A. Neuromuscular disorders and anaesthesia. Part 2: Specific neuromuscular disorders. *Continuing Education in Anaesthesia, Critical Care & Pain* 2011; 11 (4): 119–123.

12. D

Cross-clamping the aorta increases the afterload to the heart and causes a sudden increase in arterial pressure proximal to the clamp. Measures to deal with this include use of short acting vasodilators such as a GTN infusion, additional opioids, and deepening anaesthesia.

Increasing the FiO_2 is of no benefit.

Most would advocate not using the epidural until the cross clamp is removed and haemostasis achieved as hypotension could be exacerbated and more difficult to treat.

Al-Hashimi M, Thompson J. Anaesthesia for elective open abdominal aortic aneurysm repair. *Continuing Education in Anaesthesia Critical Care & Pain* 2013; 13 (6): 208–212.

13. C

The details of the case describe a patient with advanced age and comorbid disease requiring major urgent non-cardiac surgery. Based on this alone they are likely to be at high risk of perioperative death (mortality >5%) and therefore should be managed as 'high risk'. Recommendations from the National Emergency Laparotomy Audit state that objective and formal risk assessment should be carried out routinely; ASA alone is not detailed enough. Lee's revised cardiac risk index (RCRI) is more recent than Goldman's Original Cardiac Risk Index. It describes six independent risk variables for patients undergoing major non-cardiac surgery. It is validated in predicting cardiovascular risk factors only. P-POSSUM is freely available on the internet and is possibly the best validated method. Its scoring includes 12 physiological and six operative details. Hospital Episode Statistics (HES) contains details of all admissions at NHS hospitals in England and may also be linked to mortality data. APACHE II was derived in the general ICU population and is used to estimate ICU mortality.

The Royal College of Surgeons of England and Department of Health. Report on the peri-operative care of the higher risk general surgical patient 2011. Available at: https://www.rcseng.ac.uk/-/media/files/rcs/library-and-publications/non-journal-publications/higher_risk_surgical_patient_2011_web.pdf

14. D

Upper body central venous catheters (CVCs) should be positioned with the tip parallel to the vessel wall, usually in the lower superior vena cava (SVC) or the upper right atrium (RA). Common sites for tip misplacement include being too high in the superior vena cava, in the internal jugular vein, angled toward the wall of the vein, too low in the RA, in the right ventricle, in the innominate vein, and finally the subclavian vein.

Ultrasound can confirm catheter position with supraclavicular, transthoracic, and transoesophageal echocardiographic views. Electrocardiograpy and electromagnetic guidance are increasingly used to guide catheter tip positioning. Chest X-ray is most commonly used to check position due to its simplicity but cannot be described as a gold standard. Fluoroscopy with X-ray contrast in real time remains the gold standard for imaging in the difficult patient.

Association of Anaesthetists of Great Britain and Ireland. Safe vascular access 2016. *Anaesthesia* 2016; 71: 573–585.

15. B

Rivaroxaban is a direct inhibitor of factor Xa. The current guidelines suggest waiting 6 hours to commence or recommence rivaroxaban after central neuraxial block or removal of the epidural catheter to minimize the risk of vertebral canal haematoma.

It is also recommended to wait 12–18 hours after a dose of rivaroxaban before performing a central neuraxial block or removing an epidural catheter.

Davies G, Checketts MR. Regional anaesthesia and antithrombotic drugs. *Continuing Education in Anaesthesia Critical Care & Pain* 2012; 12 (1): 11–16.

Benzon HT, Avram MJ, Green D, Bonow RO. New oral anticoagulants and regional anaesthesia. *British Journal of Anaesthesia* 2013; 111 (Suppl 1): i96–i113.

16. B

The scenario describes onset features of malignant hyperthermia, a rare but life-threatening emergency. Survival depends upon early recognition and immediate management. Management is challenging due to the multiple treatments required at once and standard operating procedures with task allocation has been recommended. The highest priority in immediate management is to remove the trigger. This patient may have had suxamethonium during the RSI and is being maintained on a volatile anaesthetic agent, both of which are triggers for MH. The more insidious onset described in this case may be more in keeping the volatile as the cause.

AAGBI Safety Guideline. Malignant Hyperthermia Crisis. 2011. Available at: https://www.aagbi.org/sites/default/files/MH%20guideline%20for%20web%20v2.pdf

17. E

NICE CG 141 stipulates that haemodynamically unstable patients with UGIB should be offered OGD immediately after resuscitation and within 24 hours for all other patients. The history of alcohol excess in this patient may indicate the presence of gastro-oesophageal varices. Terlipressin is a slow sustained release synthetic analogue of vasopressin. It allows administration via intermittent injections. It reduces portal blood flow and hence variceal bleeding. It is the only vasoactive drug proven to reduce mortality. It should be given to patients with suspected variceal bleeding during resuscitation measures and prior to endoscopic confirmation. Somatostatin or octreotide can be used off licence. Erythromycin, as a prokinetic, administered prior to endoscopy may improve the chances of viewing a bleeding point but is not recommended in the current guidance.

Elsayad IA, Battu PK, Irving S. Management of acute upper GI bleeding. *BJA Education* 2017; 17 (4): 117–123.

NICE Clinical Guideline [CG 141] Acute upper gastrointestinal bleeding in over 16s: management. Published date: June 2012. Last updated: August 2016. Available at: http://www.nice.org.uk/guidance/CG141

18. D

Pre-oxygenation increases the oxygen reserve in the lungs during apnoea. End-tidal oxygen fraction ($FETO_2$) is the best marker of lung denitrogenation; an $FETO_2$ ≥0.9 is recommended. Breath-by-breath oxygen monitoring can be used to monitor the process; this should be corroborated with a capnograph as erroneous values of $FETO_2$ may be displayed because of apparatus dead space, face mask leak, and dilution from high fresh gas flows. A fresh gas flow rate of ≥10 L/min is required for effective denitrogenation, and a tight mask-to-face seal is essential to reduce air entrainment.

Difficult Airway Society. Guidelines for failed intubation in obstetrics. *Anaesthesia* 2015; 70: 1286–1306.

19. D

The PPV of a test is a proportion that is useful to clinicians because it answers the question: 'How likely is it that this patient has the disease given that the test result is positive?' In this example, there are 60 true positives and 20 false positives.

Positive predictive value = True positives/(True positives + False positives).

PPV = 60/(60 + 20) = 0.75.

Lalkhen AG, McCluskey A. Clinical tests: sensitivity and specificity. *Continuing Education in Anaesthesia, Critical Care & Pain* 2008; 8 (6): 221–223.

20. D

Urgent surgery will require safe rapid sequence intubation. Only rocuronium and succinylcholine have the rapid onset of muscular relaxation required to secure the airway. Circulating sugammadex will render rocuronium ineffective (and to a lesser extent vecuronium). Succinylcholine will be safer to use, although its effects will be prolonged and ventilatory support on ICU will be required postoperatively. We already know the intubation grade was straight forward. Rocuronium can be used again within 5 min of routine reversal with sugammadex but the dose should be 1.2 mg/kg and will take 4 min to provide relaxation (not adequate for true RSI).

Waiting times for re-administration of neuromuscular blocking agents after reversal with sugammadex are as shown in Table 6.1.

Table 6.1 Re-administration of rocuronium or vecuronium after routine reversal (up to 4 mg/kg sugammadex)

Minimum waiting time	Neuromuscular blocking agent and dose to be administered
5 min	**1.2** mg/kg rocuronium
4 hours	**0.6** mg/kg rocuronium or 0.1 mg/kg vecuronium

The onset of neuromuscular blockade may be prolonged up to approximately 4 min, and the duration of neuromuscular blockade may be shortened up to approximately 15 min after re-administration of rocuronium 1.2 mg/kg within 30 min of sugammadex administration. Based on pharmacokinetic modelling the recommended waiting time in patients with mild or moderate renal impairment for re-use of 0.6 mg/kg rocuronium or 0.1 mg/kg vecuronium after routine reversal with sugammadex should be 24 hours. If a shorter waiting time is required, the rocuronium dose for a new neuromuscular blockade should be 1.2 mg/kg.

Sugammadex data sheet. Available at: https://www.accessdata.fda.gov/drugsatfda_docs/label/2015/022225lbl.pdf

21. A

Hypoventilation is common due to increased BMI and postoperative analgesia and sedation. It improves rapidly with oxygen supplementation. Atelectasis and pulmonary micro-emboli would cause shunt in the lungs and this is not corrected by oxygen therapy. D and E are unlikely to be significant 1 hour after the procedure has finished.

Adams J. Obesity in anaesthesia and intensive care. *British Journal of Anaesthesia* 2000; 85: 91–108.

Association of Anaesthetists of Great Britain and Ireland Society for Obesity and Bariatric Anaesthesia. Perioperative management of the obese surgical patient. *Anaesthesia* 2015; 70 (7): 765–891.

22. D

Phaeochromocytoma tumours secrete a variable mixture of catecholamines and patients may present with the classic triad of headache, palpitations, and sweating. Hypertension is also present in around 90% of cases. Seven to 14 days prior to surgery patients would be established on sympathetic blockade, first alpha and then beta. In this case phenoxybenzamine and atenolol. Unopposed beta blockade is avoided due to the theoretical risk of increasing vasoconstriction by clocking beta-2 receptors. Phenoxybenzamine is a non-selective, non-competitive long-acting alpha-blocker. It is used to reduce the effects of catecholamine surges intraoperatively but may be implicated in postoperative hypotension due to its long half-life. Its action may persist beyond when the secreting tumour is devascularized. This hypotension is often resistant and primarily due to vasodilatation. Noradrenaline (norepinephrine) is used initially to provide an increase in peripheral vascular resistance. Vasopressin is a second line if hypotension remains refractory.

Connor D, Boumphrey S. Perioperative care of phaemochromocytoma. *BJA Education* 2016; 16 (5): 153–158.

23. E

The magnitude of physiological effect caused by aortic cross-clamping during surgery is influenced by how distally the clamp is applied along the course of the aorta. Perfusion to the lower half of the body is dependent on collateral circulation. Clamp application increases the systemic vascular resistance with a sudden increase in arterial blood pressure proximally. Releasing the aortic cross clamp suddenly drops systemic vascular resistance by 70–80% primarily causing hypotension. Pooling of blood in the lower half of the body, ischaemia–reperfusion injury, and the washout of anaerobic metabolites causing metabolic (lactic) acidosis all also make a contribution. This can cause direct myocardial suppression and profound peripheral vasodilatation. Coronary blood flow and left ventricular end-diastolic volume also decrease (almost 50% from pre-clamp levels) after clamp release.

Al-Hashimi M, Thompson J. Anaesthesia for elective open abdominal aortic aneurysm repair. *Continuing Education in Anaesthesia Critical Care & Pain,* 2013; 13 (6): 208–212.

24. A

Patients are at risk of developing renal impairment due to preoperative/postoperative hypotension and hypovolaemia, direct ischaemia from aortic clamping, and emboli. To avoid postoperative renal impairment, every effort should be made to maintain adequate perfusion pressure and limit the duration of suprarenal clamping. Many anaesthetists administer drugs such as mannitol, furosemide, or dopamine to prevent renal failure but there is no convincing evidence that they improve outcome. The main priority is to maintain an adequate extracellular fluid volume intra- and postoperatively.

Leonard A, Thompson J. Anaesthesia for ruptured abdominal aortic aneurysm. *Continuing Education in Anaesthesia, Critical Care & Pain* 2008; 8 (1): 11–15.

25. E.

A is incorrect; the Minto is the remifentanil model and in B the value of k_{eo} is incorrect.

Neither Marsh nor Minto models are particularly good for obese patients as they were not included in the original study. It is argued that the Marsh model is better understood and more commonly used, hence there is more experience with it making it the safer option.

Marsh does not discriminate by age, simply whether adult or not. Schnider, however, does.

Three exponential functions of infusion are the basis of TCI (most correct answer) and correspond to three theoretical body compartments.

Absalom AR, Mani V, De Smet T, Struys MMRF. Pharmacokinetic models for propofol—defining and illuminating the devil in the detail. *British Journal of Anaesthesia* 2009; 103 (1): 26– 37.

1. **A 76-year-old man requires right upper lobectomy of lung for bronchial carcinoma. He attends preoperative assessment to identify his suitability for surgery. His lung function tests reveal a forced expiratory volume in 1 second (FEV_1) of 1.3 L. The next most appropriate investigation is:**
   A. Cardiopulmonary exercise testing (CPET)
   B. 6-min walk test
   C. Arterial blood gas
   D. Calculation of predicted postoperative lung volumes
   E. Echocardiography

2. **You review a 72-year-old woman in preoperative assessment who is listed for laparoscopic cholecystectomy. She is a lifelong heavy smoker but with no significant medical history in her notes. Pulmonary function tests were ordered because of shortness of breath after one flight of stairs. The volume–time curve reaches a plateau, and expiration lasts at least 6 seconds. Repeated attempts are similar. FEV_1 is 40%, forced vital capacity (FVC) is 65% and predicted FEV_1/FVC ratio is 60%. The most likely diagnosis is:**
   A. Poor effort
   B. Normal
   C. Restrictive
   D. Obstructive
   E. Mixed

3. **A 64-year-old man undergoing transurethral resection of prostate (TURP) under spinal anaesthesia. The procedure has been going on for 90 min and the measured blood loss is 600 mL. The patient starts to complain of headache and nausea and is becoming a little agitated. His SaO$_2$ is 95% on 4 L via a Hudson mask. His blood pressure drops to 84/34 mmHg and his heart rate drops to 52 bpm. You stop the surgery. What is the most appropriate immediate pharmacological management?**

   A. Ephedrine
   B. Fluid bolus
   C. Metaraminol
   D. Furosemide
   E. Hypertonic saline

4. **A 48-year-old lady has a mastectomy with a latissimus dorsi reconstruction under general anaesthesia. She has a history of well-controlled asthma only. What is be the best strategy to preserve flap perfusion in the perioperative period?**

   A. Active warming to maintain normothermia
   B. Using isoflurane as the volatile anaesthetic agent
   C. Maintain urine output >2 mL/kg with diuretics
   D. Haemodilution to a haematocrit of 20%
   E. Phenlyephrine infusion to maintain a MAP >80 mmHg

5. **A 79-year-old patient presents for a total knee replacement. The patient has a history of stable angina and chronic obstructive pulmonary disease. You review the patient preoperatively. Which of the following is a specific indicator of frailty?**

   A. Body mass index (BMI) <25
   B. Female gender
   C. Anaemia
   D. Unintentional weight loss
   E. High pain score

6. **A 76-year-old man attends the preoperative clinic prior to elective removal of ingrown toenail under general anaesthetic. He has no significant past medical history, takes no mediation, and has good functional status. His BMI is 28. What are the most appropriate preoperative investigations?**

   A. Full blood count (FBC), urea and electrolytes (U&E), and electrocardiogram (ECG)
   B. FBC and U&E
   C. U&E only
   D. ECG only
   E. No investigations required

7. **You anaesthetize a 44-year-old lady for electroconvulsive therapy (ECT). What is the most common adverse effect following electroconvulsive therapy?**
   A. Postoperative cognitive dysfunction
   B. Myocardial ischaemia
   C. Severe myalgia
   D. Fractured bone
   E. Cardiac arrhythmia

8. **You anaesthetize a 34-year-old lady for a hysteroscopy. She has no significant past medical history and does not smoke. What is the most accurate predicted risk of her suffering postoperative nausea and vomiting (PONV)?**
   A. 10%
   B. 20%
   C. 40%
   D. 60%
   E. 80%

9. **A man with type 2 diabetes presents for varicose vein surgery on your morning list. He has taken his metformin and half his usual morning dose of long-acting insulin. His capillary blood glucose (CBG) level has been checked and is 18 mmol/L. What is the next step in this patient's management?**
   A. Start a variable rate insulin infusion and proceed
   B. Cancel his operation
   C. Check his urine for ketones
   D. Give him 0.1 units/kg insulin and proceed
   E. Give him the other half of his morning long-acting insulin dose and proceed

10. **A 21-year-old woman presents for diagnostic laparoscopy as a day case. She takes no regular medication and is a non-smoker. She has no significant past medical history. She has never had a general anaesthetic and has no significant family history of illness. Her BMI is 30. What is the single best management plan for this case?**
    A. Laryngeal mask airway (LMA), spontaneous breathing, fentanyl, cyclizine, 500 mL of Hartmann's solution
    B. Endotracheal tube (ETT), intermittent positive pressure ventilation (IPPV), morphine, ondansetron, 250 mL gelofusine bolus
    C. LMA, IPPV, IV paracetamol, metoclopramide, 500 mL Hartmann's solution
    D. ETT, IPPV, IV oxycodone, dexamethasone, 1,000 L Hartmann's solution
    E. ETT, IPPV, morphine, cyclizine, 1,000 mL sodium chloride 0.9% solution

11. **A 42-year-old woman presents for elective laparoscopic cholecystectomy for biliary colic. She has diet-controlled diabetes mellitus. Her tympanic temperature is 35.7°C preoperatively. What perioperative warming strategy is indicated?**
    A. Place foil hat and warmed blankets on patient before transfer to anaesthetic room
    B. Intraoperative forced air warming blanket
    C. Intraoperative forced air warming blanket and warmed IV fluids
    D. Preoperative forced air warming blanket continued intraoperatively
    E. Intraoperative warmed IV fluids

12. **A 52-year-old woman with chronic liver disease is listed for mastectomy for carcinoma. You see her preoperatively to discuss her risks. Which of the following variables carries the greatest operative risk?**
    A. Grade 2 encephalopathy
    B. Poorly controlled ascites
    C. Serum bilirubin of 20 mg/dL
    D. Serum albumin of 32 g/L
    E. Prothrombin time of 29 seconds

13. **A 56-year-old man presents for emergency repair of obstructed inguinal hernia. His BMI is 45 and he is being treated for hypertension. His wife reports that he snores loudly and routinely falls asleep while watching television. The best perioperative management plan is:**
    A. Proceed with general anaesthesia and ventilate for 12 hours postoperatively on ITU
    B. Proceed under spinal anaesthesia with intrathecal morphine and no systemic sedation
    C. Proceed with general anaesthesia, avoid opioids, and monitor on HDU postoperatively
    D. Proceed with general anaesthesia, titrate opioids carefully, and monitor on ITU postoperatively
    E. Proceed under field block

14. **A 65-year-old patient presents to preoperative assessment for elective total knee replacement. He has no other past medical history. He is brought to your attention as his BP is 172/105. His resting ECG and renal function are normal. The most appropriate course of action is:**
    A. Proceed to surgery
    B. Proceed to surgery, inform GP
    C. Postpone surgery, request ambulatory BP monitor
    D. Postpone surgery, recommend immediate treatment by GP
    E. Postpone surgery until BP is below 140/90

15. **A 75-year-old man presents for trans-urethral resection of prostate (TURP) for suspicion of cancer. He is on ticagrelor since having a cardiac stent inserted six months ago. He requests regional anaesthesia as he experienced significant postoperative nausea and vomiting after his last general anaesthetic. What is the best course of action?**

    A. Recommend proceeding with general anaesthesia
    B. Stop ticagrelor five days before surgery, proceed with spinal anaesthesia
    C. Stop ticagrelor five days before surgery, bridge with IV heparin, proceed with general anaesthesia
    D. Stop ticagrelor, wait 36 hours from last dose and proceed with spinal anaesthesia
    E. Proceed with spinal anaesthesia

16. **A 41-year-old woman requires drainage of Bartholin's cyst. She was diagnosed with multiple sclerosis (MS) one year ago following an episode of unilateral visual loss. She takes Tecfidera (dimethyl fumarate) twice daily and is currently asymptomatic. She is fasted, has a BMI of 28, and no reflux. The best anaesthetic technique to use for this case is:**

    A. General anaesthesia (GA) LMA spontaneous ventilation (SV)
    B. GA ETT IPPV with depolarizing muscle relaxant
    C. GA ETT IPPV with non-depolarizing muscle relaxant
    D. Caudal block
    E. Low spinal block

17. **A 36-year-old, self-employed joiner is listed for knee arthroscopy in the day surgery unit. During your anaesthetic preoperative visit he admits to smoking 20 cigarettes per day and has a chronic cough. He gives a three-day history of sore throat, croaky voice, and a runny nose. He is particularly keen to have his operation today as has arranged several work commitments to suit. The best plan is:**

    A. Proceed with spinal anaesthesia
    B. Proceed with general anaesthesia
    C. Proceed with femoral and sciatic nerve blocks
    D. Proceed with a Hunter's canal block
    E. Postpone until upper respiratory tract symptoms have resolved

18. **A 66-year-old male smoker is referred for preoperative (ramped, maximal, symptom-limited on a cycle ergometer) cardiopulmonary exercise test (CPET) prior to a gastrectomy for malignant disease. His results are shown below.**

Maximum/peak oxygen uptake (VO_2max) 12 mL/kg/min
Anaerobic threshold (AT) 9 mL/kg/min
Oxygen pulse 9 mL
Ventilatory equivalent for CO_2 (V_E/V_{CO2}) at AT 43
What is the best way to proceed in view of these test results?
A. Refer patient to smoking cessation clinic
B. Only proceed if intensive care bed available
C. Advise thoracic epidural analgesia
D. Advise the patient he is in the high-risk category
E. Advise the patient not to proceed with surgery

19. **You have a 25-year-old female patient on your elective orthopaedic list, for minor foot surgery. She has a BMI of 24, is ASA 1, fasted, and does not have reflux. You plan to use an LMA to maintain the airway. At induction you administer fentanyl 100 µg and propofol 200 mg IV. You open her mouth to insert the LMA and notice, for the first time, that she has a tongue stud** *in situ*. **The best action to take is:**
A. Wake the patient up
B. Remove the tongue stud and insert the LMA as planned
C. Leave the tongue stud in place and insert the LMA very carefully
D. Insert the LMA and then remove the tongue stud
E. Intubate the patient and then remove the tongue stud

20. **A 62-year-old female patient presents to preoperative assessment clinic prior to elective total knee arthroplasty. Her FBC reveals Hb 108 g/dL. Mean corpuscular volume (MCV), mean corpuscular haemoglobin (MCH), and ferritin are low. The correct management is:**
A. Inform GP, proceed to surgery
B. Start oral iron and recheck FBC in four weeks
C. Start oral iron and proceed to surgery
D. Give IV iron and recheck FBC in two weeks
E. Give IV iron and proceed to surgery

21. **A 53-year-old presents as a day case for scarf osteotomy. You use ultrasound-guided ankle block as your sole technique to allow early mobilization. Which nerve should you block first to establish the block quickly and efficiently?**
A. Saphenous nerve
B. Tibial nerve
C. Deep peroneal nerve
D. Superficial peroneal nerve
E. Sural nerve

22. **A 12-year-old, 80-kg boy is brought in for multiple dental extractions secondary to caries. He appears calm on pre-assessment but on arrival to the anaesthetic room becomes upset and uncooperative. His mother tries to calm him down without success and he refuses to have the procedure. The best option to manage this situation is:**

A. Ask the mother to restrain the child and commence anaesthesia

B. Do the next patient on the list while he calms down and agrees to procedure

C. Return him to the ward and give him an anxiolytic pre-med

D. Reschedule with a plan in place for preoperative behavioural strategies

E. Ask the dental surgeon to persuade him to have the procedure

23. **A 38-year-old female patient is assessed for elective laparoscopic cholecystectomy. She has a history of cystic fibrosis. She has had no recent chest infections and has chest physiotherapy performed every day by her partner. She can walk over a mile on the flat but her pace is limited. She becomes short of breath and unable to speak when walking quickly. The best test of her respiratory capacity is:**

A. Compare arterial blood gases and venous blood gases

B. Compare oxygen saturations at rest and on oxygen 2 L/min

C. A chest X-ray and clinical examination

D. CPET

E. Lung function tests including peak expiratory flow rate (PEFR), FEV_1, FVC, and spirometry

24. **The use of CPET in preoperative assessment can reliably predict:**

A. If patient has adequate reserve capacity

B. If invasive monitoring required perioperatively

C. If needs to be nursed in critical care postoperatively

D. Mortality rate

E. Suitability for an enhanced recovery programme

25. **A 76-year-old man requires a trans-urethral resection of the prostate (TURP). His past medical history includes stable angina, hiatus hernia, hypertension, and Alzheimer's disease. His current medication includes aspirin, ramipril, bendroflumethiazide, nicorandil, GTN spray, omeprazole, and donezepil. What is the best approach perioperatively regarding his Alzheimer's disease treatment?**

A. Stop his donezepil for two weeks prior to surgery

B. Withhold his donezepil on the morning of surgery

C. Continue his donezepil and avoid suxamethonium

D. Continue his donezepil and avoid non-depolarizing neuromuscular blockers

E. Continue his donezepil and use spinal anaesthesia

1. D

Both the British Thoracic Society (BTS) and American College of Chest Physicians (ACCP) have
produced management algorithms which are similar. The flow chart shown is an amalgamation of
the BTS and ACCP guidelines (see Figure 7.1).

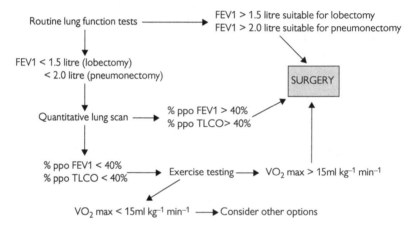

Figure 7.1 Preoperative evaluation before lung resection

Source data from: *Chest*, 123, Beckles MA, Spiro SG, Colice GL, Rudd RM, The physiogic evaluation of patients with lung cancer
being considered for resectional surgery, pp. 1055–1145, 2003; *Chest*, 123, Datta D, Lahiri B, Preoperative evaluation of patients
undergoing lung resection surgery, pp. 2096–2103, 2003.

The initial screening tool prior to lung surgery is pulmonary function tests. A measured FEV_1 >2
L is required for pneumonectomy and >1.5 L for lobectomy. If there is no comorbidity, achieving
the appropriate lung volume is sufficient. When these threshold lung volumes are not met, full
respiratory function testing allows calculation of the predicted postoperative (PPO) FEV_1 and
diffusing capacity of the lungs for carbon monoxide (DLCO). For lobectomy, the simple calculation
uses the number of bronchopulmonary segments removed compared with the total number (19)
in both lungs. In this case a right upper lobe removal carries 3/19 segments. If either (or both) the
PPO, FEV_1, or DLCO is <40%, the patient should then undergo formal CPET. The threshold VO_2
max of 15 mL/kg/min delineates between high- and medium-risk patients.

Gould G. Pearce A. Assessment of suitability for lung resection. *Continuing Education in Anaesthesia and
Critical Care and Pain* 2006; 6 (3): 97–100.

2. E

The FEV_1/FVC ratio is low (<70%) indicating obstruction. The FVC is also low indicating restriction. The results are valid as the patient has reproduced the same values on repeated blows and is able to reach plateau. In a pure restrictive disorder, the FEV_1 and FVC are both reduced to <80% but the FEV_1/FVC ratio would be >70%.

Bellamy D. *Spirometry in Practice: A practical Guide to Using Spirometry in Primary Care*, 2nd Edition. London: The BTS COPD Consortium 2005.

3. A

This clinical picture is suggestive of mild to moderate TURP syndrome. The prolonged procedure and moderate blood loss, implying a large number of open veins, are risk factors for absorption of irrigating fluid. The most important initial management is to abandon the surgery and stop intravenous fluid administration.

The syndrome is secondary to excess absorption of irrigating fluid with acute changes in intravascular volume and plasma osmolality, as well as the direct effects of glycine if it has been used.

Ephedrine would increase the heart rate and blood pressure through its alpha and beta agonist effects. Metaraminol may worsen the bradycardia.

If the situation progresses the patient may well need airway support and cardiovascular support with vasopressors. If neurological symptoms deteriorate and seizures occur, the appropriate treatment would be benzodiazepines and magnesium. Blood should be checked urgently for sodium, osmolality, and haemoglobin levels.

Diuretics are only recommended if there is acute pulmonary oedema as furosemide can worsen hyponatraemia.

Hypertonic saline is only indicated if there is severe hyponatraemia.

O'Donnell AM, Foo ITH. Anaesthesia for transurethral resection of the prostate. *Continuing Education in Anaesthesia Critical Care & Pain* 2009; 9 (3): 92–96.

4. A

Normothermia should be maintained with active warming before the start of induction of anaesthesia. Hypothermia causes vasoconstriction and increases plasma viscosity, which decrease microcirculatory flow.

Isoflurane may offer an advantage because it causes some vasodilatation and causes minimal cardiac depression but this is of less importance than good temperature control and optimal fluid balance.

Aiming for a urine output of 1–2 mL/kg is appropriate but is best achieved with goal directed fluid management rather than diuretics as volume depletion can compromise the free flap.

Isovolaemic haemodilution to achieve a haematocrit of 30–35% (0.3–0.35) improves flow by decreasing plasma viscosity. Larger reductions than this risk oxygen delivery with no further advantage in flow.

Vasoconstrictors such as noradrenaline (norepinephrine) should be avoided.

Adams J, Charlton P. Anaesthesia for microvascular free tissue transfer. *BJA CEPD Reviews* 2003; 3 (2): 33–37.

Nimalan N, Alexandre Branford O, Stocks G. Anaesthesia for free flap breast reconstruction. *BJA Education* 2016; 16 (5): 162–166.

5. D

All the other options may also be present in someone with frailty, but only unintentional weight loss is scored on *both* the frailty phenotype model and the frailty index scale.

Most frailty definitions include reduced muscle strength, unintentional weight loss, tiredness and fatigue, and low physical activity with slow walking. These factors are scored to indicate a frailty phenotype.

The Edmonton Frail Scale assesses nine criteria to give a score: mood, cognition, general health, functional status, social support, nutrition especially history of weight loss, medication use, continence, and functional performance. This can be performed preoperatively at the bedside.

Many factors increase the risk of frailty including female sex, multiple comorbidities, low socio-economic class, depression, disability, cognitive decline, and polypharmacy. Frailty increases postoperative complications and the length of hospital stay. It can also affect the discharge destination of the patient.

Alcock M. Frailty and the peri-operative period. *Anaesthesia Tutorial of the Week* 236. Available at: http://www.frca.co.uk/Documents/236%20Frailty%20in%20anaesthesia.pdf

Griffiths R, Mehta M. Frailty and anaesthesia: what we need to know. *Continuing Education in Anaesthesia Critical Care & Pain* 2014; 14 (6): 273–277.

6. E

NICE guidance: NG45—Routine preoperative tests for elective surgery (http://nice.org.uk/guidance/ng45). This guideline covers routine preoperative tests for people aged over 16 who are having elective surgery. It prompts assessment of the patient's comorbidity versus the severity of surgery planned. It aims to reduce unnecessary testing by advising which tests to offer people before minor, intermediate, and major or complex surgery, taking into account specific comorbidities (cardiovascular, renal, and respiratory conditions, and diabetes and obesity). There is a general trend to try and reduce the volume of preoperative investigations with an emphasis on individual assessment. This patient has an ASA class of 1 and is having minor (or severity grade 1) surgery. While the age is increased, guidance suggests that this in isolation does not necessitate testing. Patients with significant comorbidity requiring intermediate/major surgery will have basic tests routinely performed.

The AAGBI Safety Guideline. Preoperative Assessment and Patient Preparation, the Role of the Anaesthetist (2010) https://www.aagbi.org/sites/default/files/preop2010.pdf is an older guideline which suggests patients >80 years should have ECG but also recognizes the suggestion that patients of any age with no major comorbidities (ASA physical status 1 or 2) presenting for day surgery may not need any preoperative investigations.

7. A

Disorientation, impaired attention, and memory problems are frequent post-ictally and short-term memory impairment lasting several weeks occurs in more than 50% of patients.

ECT causes activation of the autonomic nervous system. Initially there is a short parasympathetic discharge associated with bradycardia and hypotension. A more prominent sympathetic response follows with increased BP, heart rate, and myocardial oxygen consumption. This may be associated occasionally with cardiac arrhythmias and myocardial ischaemia and infarction particularly if there is pre-existing disease.

Historically during unmodified fits (i.e. without a GA) there was a high incidence of fractures and dislocations but these are now rare.

Myalgia either from seizure activity or succinylcholine can occur but symptoms are usually mild.

Gratrix AP, Enright SM. Epilepsy in anaesthesia and intensive care. *Continuing Education in Anaesthesia Critical Care & Pain* 2005; 5 (4): 118–121.

8. C

There are two simplified PONV scores for adults—the Koivurata et al. and the Apfel et al. scores. Both would count female gender and non-smoking status as risk factors giving a predicted incidence of approximately 40%.

In the Apfel score when 0, 1, 2, 3, or 4 factors are present, the risk of PONV is 10%, 20%, 40%, 60%, and 80% respectively. The four risk factors in the Apfel scoring system are female gender, non-smoking status, history of PONV or motion sickness, and postoperative use of opioids in the Apfel scoring system.

The Koivurata system gives a score of 1 for the five risk factors of female gender, non-smoking status, history of PONV, history of motion sickness, and duration of surgery >60 min. If 0, 1, 2, 3, 4, or 5 risk factors are present the incidence of PONV is 17%, 18%, 42%, 54%, 74%, and 87% respectively.

Pierre S, Whelan R. Nausea and vomiting after surgery. *Continuing Education in Anaesthesia Critical Care & Pain*, 2013; 13 (1) 28–32.

9. C

It is important to maintain good glycaemic control aiming for a CBG level of 6–10 mmol/L in diabetic patients. Studies have shown that a high preoperative and perioperative glucose and HbA1c levels are associated with poor surgical outcomes in both the elective and emergency situations. There is increased risk of postoperative respiratory, urinary tract, and surgical site infections, and increased risk of myocardial infarction and acute kidney injury.

If the glucose level exceeds 12 mmol/L it is important to rule out diabetic ketoacidosis (DKA) which is a medical emergency. If DKA is not present you should treat the hyperglycaemia with insulin as a bolus initially but if blood glucose remains difficult to control with a variable rate infusion. Once blood glucose has normalized surgery could proceed.

AAGBI Peri-operative management of the surgical patient with diabetes 2015. Available at: https://www.aagbi.org/sites/default/files/Diabetes%20FINAL%20published%20in%20Anaesthesia%20Sept%2015%20with%20covers%20for%20online[1].pdf

10. D

Rationale: Answers ordered in: Airway/Ventilation/Analgesia/Antiemesis/Fluids

In terms of airway control, obese, pneumoperitoneum, Trendelenburg tilt, possible lithotomy all point to definitive airway in the hands of ST3/4 trainee (NAP 4). Therefore A and C excluded.

Young, female, non-smoker for day case, therefore PONV prophylaxis and *adequate* analgesia paramount.

B and E both have morphine, cyclizine has sedative side effects, 250 mL Gelofusine is a resuscitation fluid prescription, not replacement.

11. D

This is an elective procedure and her temperature is less than 36.0°C, hence preoperative active warming is recommended until temperature exceeds 36.0°C.

Forced air warming is indicated intraoperatively because having hypothermia preoperatively and a total anaesthetized time likely to be greater than 30 min are both independent indications and also meets criteria equating to 'high risk' of intraoperative hypothermia (high risk is having at least two factors from the following list: ASA II-V, hypothermia preoperatively, combined GA and RA, at risk of cardiovascular complications and having intermediate or major level surgery).

Warmed IV fluids are not specifically recommended unless over 500 mL has been infused.

Passive measures such as foil hats and warmed blankets will only prevent further heat loss and will not correct existing hypothermia.

NICE guideline Inadvertent Perioperative Hypothermia. An integrated View on all NICE has said regarding inadvertent preoperative hypothermia. Available at: https://pathways.nice.org.uk/pathways/inadvertent-perioperative-hypothermia.

12. B

Using the Pugh modification of Child's criteria points are given for increasing abnormality of encephalopathy, ascites, serum bilirubin, serum albumin, and prothrombin time. The greater the abnormality, the greater the score. These are added together to predict operative mortality risk.

Vaja R, McNicol L, Sisleyl. Anaesthesia for patients with liver disease. *Continuing Education in Anaesthesia Critical Care & Pain* 2010; 10 (1): 15–19.

13. D

Using the STOP-BANG score, the patient scores over 5 therefore is at high risk of having obstructive sleep apnoea (OSA) and episodes of postoperative desaturation and hypoxaemia following the emergency procedure.

Spinal anaesthesia is not usually a good option in the obstructed patient, and the incidence of respiratory complications in OSA from intrathecal opioids is largely unknown, and thus poses a risk to the patient.

The cumulative sedative nature of anaesthesia and analgesics should be minimized and therefore it would not be optimal to electively ventilate the patient.

Field block will be inadequate for this emergency case. It is likely that some opioid will be required for the procedure and also to help maintain a steady blood pressure during intubation and extubation. OSA is made worse by general anaesthesia as well as opioid analgesics so while monitoring on HDU may be adequate, monitoring saturation on ITU postoperatively is ideal, in case advanced airway and ventilation support becomes necessary.

Orlov D, Ankichetty S, Chung F, Brull R. Cardiorespiratory complications of neuraxial opioids in patients with obstructive sleep apnea: A systematic review. *Journal of Clinical Anesthesia* 2013; 25 (7): 591–599.

14. B

Preoperative assessment clinics should measure the blood pressures of patients who present without documentation of primary care blood pressures. If the blood pressure is raised above 180 mmHg systolic or 110 mmHg diastolic, the patient should return to their general practice for primary care assessment and management of their blood pressure. If the blood pressure is above 140 mmHg systolic or 90 mmHg diastolic, but below 180 mmHg systolic and below 110 mmHg diastolic, the GP should be informed, but elective surgery should not be postponed according to AAGBI/British Hypertensive Society guidance.

Hartle A, McCormack T, Carlisle J, et al. The measurement of adult blood pressure and management of hypertension before elective surgery. Joint Guidelines from the Association of Anaesthetists of Great Britain and Ireland and the British Hypertension Society. *Anaesthesia* 2016; 71 (3): 326–327.

15. B

Ticagrelor is a platelet adenosine diphosphate (ADP) P_2Y12 receptor inhibitor. Its antiplatelet effect can be removed by stopping the drug and waiting. Ticagrelor is a longer acting drug with a half life of 18 hours and it is recommended waiting five days from the last dose before performing spinal anaesthesia. Bridging with heparin is not necessary in this case as antiplatelet therapy can be safely discontinued at six months with bare metal stents. The stents with have epithelialized by this time and the risk of thrombosis is no longer increased.

Regional anaesthesia and patients with abnormalities of coagulation OAA and AAGBI 2013. Available at: https://www.aagbi.org/sites/default/files/rapac_2013_web.pdf

Wallentin L. P2Y12 inhibitors: differences in properties and mechanisms of action and potential consequences for clinical use. *European Heart Journal* 2009; 30 (16): 1964–1977.

16. A

This is a case of keeping it simple and not overcomplicating matters. General anaesthesia *per se* does not precipitate any deterioration or relapse of multiple sclerosis. (However, a major stress response to extensive surgery may well do.) Induction agents, volatiles, and relaxants are known to be safe.

With a BMI of 28 the patient is suitable for anaesthetizing using a laryngeal airway (fasted, no reflux) because it is a very short procedure. She could also be intubated and ventilated with or without muscle relaxants, paying attention to elapsed time prior to reversal and safe extubation.

Regional anaesthesia is thought to be safe although there may be an increased blood–brain barrier permeability and sensitivity to CNS toxicity with MS. It is prudent to use the minimum dose possible of local anaesthetic. Some related hypotension has been considered relatively resistant to vasopressors.

A low spinal block would be more appropriate than a caudal (density, predictability, ease of siting, reliability) but would outlast this operation significantly.

Tecfidera (dimethyl fumarate) is one of several disease modifying treatments for MS. It requires no special precautions to be taken with drugs used in anaesthesia including muscle relaxants.

Kyttä J, Rosenberg PH. Anaesthesia for patients with multiple sclerosis. *Annales Chirurgiae et Gynaecologiae* 1984; 73(5): 299–303.

17. A

You can proceed with spinal anaesthesia. The risks of proceeding with symptoms of upper respiratory tract infection versus postponing the procedure at great inconvenience to the patient must be balanced pragmatically. There are no systemic signs of illness and his symptoms are all localized 'above the clavicles'. The risks of general anaesthesia may outweigh the benefit of proceeding but short effective spinal anaesthesia can be achieved in a day surgery setting. Prilocaine is often used in this situation.

Femoral and sciatic blocks take some time to perform and develop. Their duration of action is at least 12 hours and it is not ideal to send a patient home with a numb leg. A Hunter's canal block alone will not provide adequate anaesthesia for a knee arthroscopy.

Bhatia N, Barber N. Dilemmas in the preoperative assessment of children. *Continuing Education in Anaesthesia Critical Care & Pain* 2011; 11 (6) 214–218.

Fennelly ME, Hall GM. Anaesthesia and upper respiratory tract infections—A non-existent hazard? *British Journal of Anaesthesia* 1990; 64 (5): 535–536.

18. D

CPET testing helps inform perioperative management of individual patients by allocating them to a high- or low-risk category for postoperative morbidity and mortality.

This patients results place him very clearly into the high risk group; his VO_2 max and anaerobic threshold (AT) are well below the values accepted as inferring low risk (18 mL/kg/min and 14 mL/kg/min respectively).

Following this risk assessment, the patient and surgeon/anaesthetist team can put plans in place to minimize post-operative risks by instituting a variety of appropriate measures. Such measures may include higher levels of monitoring, particular forms of analgesia and higher level of monitoring in the postoperative period. These specifics are decided on a patient to patient basis and are not mandated by the test results.

Smoking cessation would improve the test results but surgery for malignant disease should not be unduly postponed for this reason.

Moran J, Wilson F, Guinan E, et al. Role of cardiopulmonary exercise testing as a risk-assessment method in patients undergoing intra-abdominal surgery: A systematic review. *British Journal of Anaesthesia* 2016; 116 (2): 177–191.

Richardson K, Levett DZH, Jack S, Grocott MPW. Fit for surgery? Perspectives on preoperative exercise testing and training. *British Journal of Anaesthesia* 2017; 119 (Suppl 1): i34–i43,

19. A

Waking the patient up is the safest action to take, bearing in mind the case can be rescheduled. While many would be tempted to leave the tongue stud in place and proceed carefully with the LMA (answer C), this confers potential risks including bleeding, oedema, and a can't intubate, can't ventilate (CICV) scenario (see the references below).

Intubation requires instrumentation of the tongue and carries risks of its own both at induction and emergence.

The danger in removing the tongue stud after induction but before insertion of an airway device is that can fall or be dropped into the airway. Removal of a slippery stud on a mobile tongue whilst wearing gloves is tricky. Removing the tongue stud with the LMA *in situ* does not protect the airway as the seal of the LMA may not cover the entire glottic opening.

There is an additional possibility that if the patient has concealed details of her piercings, there may be further inaccuracies in her pre-operative assessment.

DeBoer S, McNeil M, Amundson T. Body piercing and airway management: photo guide to tongue jewelry removal techniques. *AANA Journal* 2008; 76 (1): 19–23.

Kuczkowski KM, Benumof JL. Tongue piercing and obstetric anesthesia: Is there cause for concern? *Journal of Clinical Anaesthesia* 2002; 14 (6): 447–448.

20. B

The blood results indicate iron deficiency anaemia. The haemoglobin level should be optimized preoperatively to reduce the likelihood of perioperative transfusion. IV iron is not indicated first line in elective non-cancer surgery where there is no obvious requirement to rapidly improve the preoperative haemoglobin. Response to oral iron should be confirmed before proceeding with rechecking of FBC.

Evans C. Preoperative anaemia management. Royal College of Anaesthetists. 2016. Available at: https://www.rcoa.ac.uk/sites/default/files/POM-DrEvans.pdf

Hans GA, Jones N. Preoperative anaemia. *Continuing Education in Anaesthesia Critical Care & Pain* 2013; 13 (3): 71–74.

Muñoz M, Acheson A, Auerbach M, et al. International consensus statement on the peri-operative management of anaemia and iron deficiency. *Anaesthesia* 2017; 72: 233–247.

21. B

All five nerves, the tibial, deep and superficial peroneal, sural, and saphenous, are blocked in an ankle block. The tibial nerve should be blocked first because it is the largest and therefore it takes the longest time for the block to develop.

Purushothaman L, Allan AGL, Bedforth N. Ultrasound-guided ankle block. *Continuing Education in Anaesthesia Critical Care & Pain* 2013; 13 (5): 174–178.

22. D

Preoperative anxiety is common in children and young adults and is associated with adverse clinical outcomes. A 12-year-old boy of average intelligence can give or withhold consent. Physical restraint is not an option for older children. Measures to reduce anxiety include sedative premedication, behavioural/play therapy, and presence of parent in the anaesthetic room. Sedative premedication also requires a degree of willing and consent from the child and the present situation may be too fraught to explain and deliver this. Behavioural therapy is time consuming and there is no evidence to support that having a parent in the anaesthetic room does reduce anxiety in a child, though this remains hotly debated.

Waiting for the patient to calm down is unlikely to be successful and along with persuasion by the dentist, provides no guarantee of compliance in the anaesthetic room.

O'Sullivan M, Wong GK. Preinduction techniques to relieve anxiety in children undergoing general anaesthesia. *Continuing Education in Anaesthesia Critical Care & Pain* 2013; 13 (6): 196–199.

23. E

From the question we can ascertain the patient has limited exercise capacity. FEV_1 is an important indicator of ability to cough and engage successfully with physiotherapy postoperatively. Lung function tests showing a reduction in FEV_1 to <1 L/min may indicate the need for postoperative ventilation.

CPET primarily categorizes patients into high or low risk of postoperative complications.

Fitzgerald M, Ryan D. Cystic fibrosis and anaesthesia. *Continuing Education in Anaesthesia Critical Care & Pain* 2011; 11 (6): 204–209.

24. A

CPET testing is an accessible, minimally invasive test of the patient's exercise capacity. This reflects the cardiorespiratory demands that will be made of the body during, and for some time after, major surgery. The information can help with planning appropriate perioperative care for individual patients.

Following the exercise test and recovery period, the cardiorespiratory variables measured are analysed taking into consideration any significant external factors. The results are provided to the referring clinician advising whether the patient is deemed to be at high risk or low risk of perioperative morbidity and mortality. It is then the decision of the referring clinician and the surgical team how best to manage the patient in view of this result. The CPET results do not mandate whether or not surgery should proceed, nor do they advise upon need for intensive care or high dependency availability or the best techniques to be used.

UCL Centre for Anaesthesia Critical Care and Pain Medicine CPET test. Available at: https://www.ucl.ac.uk/anaesthesia/research/CPET

25 E

Donezepil is an anti-cholinesterase used in the treatment of dementia. It can potentially prolong the effect of depolarizing neuromuscular blockers and decrease or reverse the effects of non-depolarizing neuromuscular blockers. Some guidelines recommend stopping anticholinesterase agents before elective surgery but donezepil has a long half-life of 70 hours and would require a washout period of two to three weeks. A prolonged period without this treatment may lead to an irreversible decline in cognitive function. Therefore, option E offers the best perioperative anaesthetic option by avoiding a general anaesthetic and potential for drug interaction. It would also have the beneficial effect of reducing the risk of the patient developing postoperative delirium.

Alcorn S, Foo I. Perioperative management of patients with dementia. *BJA Education* 2017; 17 (3): 94–98.

1. **Regarding the measurement of blood pressure in an adult with a sphygmomanometer, the systolic and diastolic pressures respectively are best indicated by which Korotkov sounds?**
   A. I and II
   B. I and IV
   C. I and V
   D. II and IV
   E. II and V

2. **A 62-year-old man is managed in cardiac intensive care with cardiogenic shock following acute myocardial infarction. He has oliguria, raised lactate, and altered mental status. Which of the following is an absolute contraindication to the use of an intra-aortic balloon pump?**
   A. Aortic regurgitation
   B. Uncontrolled sepsis
   C. Tachyarrhythmia
   D. Peripheral vascular disease
   E. Abdominal aortic aneurysm

3. **The most accurate means of measuring cardiac output is:**
   A. Pulse contour analysis LiDCO
   B. Echocardiography
   C. Thoracic bio-impedance
   D. Oesophageal Doppler
   E. Pulmonary artery catheter

4. **Regarding paravertebral block, the most common complication is:**
   A. Pneumothorax
   B. Hypotension
   C. Vascular puncture
   D. Dural puncture
   E. Block failure

5. **A 68-year-old lady presents for an emergency laparotomy for a suspected viscus perforation. She has chronic moderate mitral regurgitation. What is the most important haemodynamic goal in her perioperative management?**
   A. Keep pulmonary vascular resistance as low as possible
   B. Maintain forward flow through the heart
   C. Aim to reduce preload to the heart
   D. Aim for a slow normal heart rate
   E. Use vasoconstrictors to increase systemic vascular resistance

6. **You anaesthetize a 61-year-old lady for a coronary artery bypass graft. She is on aspirin and clopidogrel following a myocardial infarction three months ago. You intend to monitor her coagulation status using thromboelastography. Which of these statements most accurately describes the use of a viscoelastic point-of care device?**
   A. It will reflect the effects of hypothermia
   B. It will demonstrate the effects of aspirin
   C. It will demonstrate the effects of clopidogrel
   D. It can guide the administration of specific blood products
   E. It is more cost effective than conventional laboratory tests

7. **A 28-year-old man is in the Emergency Department resuscitation room. He was the driver of a car involved in a head on collision at 40 mph. He has no significant past medical history. You carry out the primary survey. Which potential injury on primary survey is the most** *immediately* **life threatening?**
   A. Myocardial contusion
   B. Pulmonary contusion
   C. Massive haemothorax
   D. Diaphragmatic rupture
   E. Traumatic aortic injury

8. **A 59-year-old man is in Intensive Care with severe cardiogenic shock following a massive myocardial infarction. He has not responded to initial treatment with inotropes so an intra-aortic balloon pump (IABP) is inserted. What is the most common side effect of IABP insertion?**
   A. Aortic dissection
   B. Iliac dissection
   C. Infective endocarditis
   D. Aortic perforation
   E. Limb ischaemia

9. **A two-year-old child undergoes elective cardiac surgery to correct a large ventricular septal defect (VSD). Intravenous induction of anaesthesia commences with fentanyl, propofol, and pancuronium. The child is intubated correctly and uneventfully but becomes cyanotic soon after induction despite high concentrations of oxygen. What is the most appropriate initial action?**

   A. Hyperventilation, phenylephrine bolus
   B. Hyperventilation, propofol bolus
   C. Hypoventilation, increase positive end-expiratory pressure (PEEP), 8% sevoflurane
   D. Hyperventilation, increase PEEP, propofol bolus
   E. Hypoventilation, phenylephrine bolus

10. **A 59-year-old man with dilated cardiomyopathy presents as an emergency with an incarcerated inguinal hernia. His medication incudes carvedilol, lisinopril, and furosemide. He reports shortness of breath on exertion and ankle swelling. What is the most important cardiovascular goal in the anaesthetic management of this patient?**

    A. Increase afterload
    B. Avoid inotropes
    C. Avoid bradycardia
    D. Maintain sinus rhythm
    E. Increase preload

11. **You assess a 70-year-old lady for a left total knee replacement. She has hypertension, osteoarthritis, and a pacemaker. Her pacemaker card confirms the pacemaker is DDD. Which of the following best explains what DDD means?**

    A. Direct pacing of ventricle with dual response
    B. Direct pacing of atrium with dual response
    C. Direct sensing of the atrium with ventricular pacing
    D. Direct pacing of both atrium and ventricle with antitachycardia function
    E. Pacing and sensing of both atrium and ventricle with dual response

12. **A 70-year-old man has been diagnosed with bronchial cancer in his left lower lobe. He is being investigated and pre-assessed for a lobectomy. Which result from his investigations would indicate he is potentially unsuitable for surgery?**

    A. An FEV_1 of 1.1 L
    B. VO_{2max} of 25 mL/min
    C. Predicted postoperative FEV_1 of 50%
    D. Arterial $PaCO_2$ of 6.5 kPA
    E. Oxygen saturation on room air of 91%

13. **You anaesthetize a 62-year-old man for a laparoscopic hernia repair. He had a cardiac transplant three years ago and has been stable since then. During the procedure, his heart rate drops to 37 bpm and his blood pressure falls to 81/56 mmHg. This does not improve despite the surgeon deflating the pneumo-peritoneum. What is the most appropriate management?**
    A. Administer ephedrine
    B. Administer glycopyrrolate
    C. Administer atropine
    D. Administer metaraminol
    E. Administer hydralazine

14. **A 58-year-old man requires elective left thoracotomy for lung resection. He is a smoker with moderate COPD. He has no other significant past medical history. His platelet count and coagulation screen are normal. What is the best choice of postoperative pain relief?**
    A. Paravertebral block
    B. Multimodal analgesia
    C. Thoracic epidural
    D. IV opioids
    E. Intercostal nerve blocks

15. **A 72-year-old man presents for a coronary artery bypass graft. You use the EURO Score II to determine his operative risk during your pre-assessment. Which of these factors conveys the highest risk?**
    A. Emergency surgery
    B. Ejection fraction <20%
    C. Age >60
    D. Chronic lung disease
    E. A myocardial infarction 70 days ago

16. **A 54-year-old man is undergoing bronchoscopy and biopsy of bronchial tumour. During the procedure haemorrhage occurs and results in an emergency thoracotomy. You had consented him for postoperative patient-controlled analgesia (PCA) morphine in your preoperative assessment. The best action would be to:**
    A. Perform thoracic epidural at the end of the operation while still under general anaesthesia (GA)
    B. Perform thoracic epidural at the end of the operation once patient awake
    C. Perform a paravertebral block in addition to the PCA morphine
    D. Give PCA morphine only as per preoperative plan
    E. Keep sedated and ventilated on Intensive Care

17. **A 55-year-old patient requires an elective left pneumonectomy for primary lung malignancy. What is the best choice of endotracheal tube?**
    A. Uncut standard endotracheal tube
    B. Cut standard endotracheal tube and bronchial blocker
    C. Left-sided double lumen tube
    D. Right-sided double lumen tube
    E. Reinforced endotracheal tube

18. **A 55-year-old man presents to A&E with sudden onset pleuritic chest pain and reduced air entry in his right hemithorax. He has no shortness of breath, all vital signs are normal, and he appears otherwise well. He has no other past medical history. He is a current smoker of 20 cigarettes/day for the last 15 years. A 1.5-cm pneumothorax rim is diagnosed on chest X-ray. The recommended management is:**
    A. Insert chest drain
    B. Inpatient observation only
    C. High flow oxygen therapy and inpatient observation
    D. Aspirate pneumothorax
    E. Discharge with advice to return if symptomatic

19. **You anaesthetize a 68-year-old man for open left-sided pneumonectomy. He is positioned in the right lateral position. Before the start of the procedure you notice a sudden increase in airway pressure from 25 cmH$_2$O to 45 cmH$_2$O. The best action to take is:**
    A. Pass a suction catheter down the endotracheal tube
    B. Check muscle relaxation with peripheral nerve stimulator
    C. Observe capnography trace
    D. Check the tube position with a fibrescope
    E. Auscultate the chest

20. **You are comparing pressure–volume curves in asthmatic patients during an acute asthma attack and comparing it with healthy subjects. Which of the following observed differences is the best indicator of the increased work of breathing in the patients with asthma?**
    A. Larger hysteresis loop
    B. Longer expiratory time
    C. Pressure–volume curve starts at a higher end-expiratory pressure
    D. Slope of the inspiratory limb is initially less steep
    E. Tidal volume is smaller

1. C

Phase I is the first appearance of sound which indicates the systolic. Phase IV is the abrupt muffling of sounds that was previously used for estimation of the diastolic. More recently there has been a move towards using phase V (silence) instead to indicate the diastolic as this is more reproducible and less amenable to interobserver variation.

Ward M, Langton JA. Blood pressure measurement. *Continuing Education in Anaesthesia Critical Care & Pain* 2007; 7 (4): 122–126.

2. A.

Aortic regurgitation is the only absolute contraindication as the presence of the IABP worsens the magnitude of regurgitation, particularly undesirable when the left ventricle is failing.

Krishna M, Zacharowski K. Principles of intra-aortic balloon pump counterpulsation. *Continuing Education in Anaesthesia Critical Care & Pain* 2009; 9 (1): 24–28.

3. E

A pulmonary artery catheter (PAC) with thermodilution is the gold standard monitor to measure cardiac output. It is currently out of favour outside specialist centres due to the skill required for correct positioning and the increased risk of major complications. A search for less or non-invasive cardiac output monitoring has led to the advent of many new devices. However they are subject to varied areas of error/estimation leading to potential problems with accuracy. A PAC remains the standard against which other less invasive monitors are measured.

Drummond KE, Murphy E. Minimally invasive cardiac output monitors. *Continuing Education in Anaesthesia, Critical Care & Pain* 2012; 12 (1): 5–10.

4. E

The failure rate of paravertebral block in experienced hands is quoted between 6.8% and 10% which his broadly similar to epidural failure rates. Specifically reported complications include hypotension 4.6%, vascular puncture 3.8%, pleural puncture 1.1%, and pneumothorax 5.5%. The risk of complications resulting in long-term morbidity are exceedingly low.

Tighe SQM, Greene MD, Rajadurai N. Paravertebral block. *Continuing Education in Anaesthesia Critical Care & Pain* 2010; 10 (5): 133–137.

5. B

For regurgitant lesions the haemodynamic goals are 'full, fast, and forward'.

Keeping pulmonary vascular resistance as low as possible will help this but can only be achieved by avoiding hypoxia, hypercarbia, and acidosis.

Decreased arterial pressure should be treated with fluids and elevating the heart rate. A high normal heart rate of 80–100 reduces filling time of left ventricle reducing ventricular overload and encouraging forward flow. Keeping the patient well filled also promotes forward flow.

Vasoconstrictors can be used with care.

Holmes K, Gibbison B, Vohra HA. Mitral valve and mitral valve disease. *BJA Education* 2017; 17 (1): 1–9.

6. D

Thromboelastography (TEG) and rotational thromboelastometry (ROTEM) are visco-elastic point-of-care devices providing rapid bedside assessment of the overall coagulation status of the patient. Derived parameters can guide the administration of specific blood products.

Their tracings are insensitive to aspirin and clopidogrel and are poor at detecting conditions affecting platelet adhesion such as Von Willebrand's disease.

It will not reflect the effects of hypothermia as the measurement is undertaken at 37°C.

It is currently more expensive that conventional testing.

Srivastava A, Kelleher A. Point-of-care coagulation testing, *Continuing Education in Anaesthesia Critical Care & Pain.* 2013; 13 (1): 12–16.

7. C

The brief description indicates a high energy impact which raises suspicion of significant injury. Principles of management are in keeping with the advanced trauma life support doctrine of primary and secondary surveys with definitive management. The primary survey focuses on the airway, breathing, circulation, disability, and exposure (ABCDE) principle. This is conducted simultaneously with resuscitation of vital functions as set out in the Advanced Trauma Life Support Manual. The immediately life-threatening injuries identified and treated on primary survey are in the left-hand column in Table 8.1 and are indicated by the acronym ATOM-FC.

Table 8.1 Life-threatening injuries resulting from blunt force thoracic trauma

Immediate life-threatening injuries	Potentially life-threatening injuries
Airway obstruction	Traumatic aortic injury
Tension pneumothorax	Pulmonary contusion
Open pneumothorax	Myocardial contusion
Massive haemothorax	Diaphragmatic rupture
Flail chest	Oesophageal rupture
Cardiac tamponade	Tracheobronchial rupture

All of these injuries are severe and in keeping with major thoracic blunt force trauma. The most immediate life-threatening injury is massive haemothorax requiring chest drain insertion and thoracotomy if persistent.

Saayman AG, Findlay GP. The management of blunt thoracic trauma. *BJA CEPD Reviews* 2003; 3 (6): 171–174.

8. E

All of the above are possible complications but limb ischaemia is the most common. Limb ischaemia can usually be resolved by repositioning or removal of the balloon.

ATOTW 220. Intra-aortic balloon pump. Available from; http://www.frca.co.uk

Krishna M, Zacharowski K. Principles of intra-aortic balloon pump counterpulsation. *Continuing Education in Anaesthesia Critical Care & Pain* 2009; 9 (1): 24–28.

9. A

Blood flow to the lungs and body is a balance between systemic vascular resistance (SVR) and pulmonary vascular resistance (PVR). Examples of children with balanced circulation physiology who may present to local hospitals are infants with a large unrepaired atrioventricular septal defect or VSD. These infants have predominantly left-to-right shunt flow. High concentrations of oxygen will increase pulmonary blood flow (PBF) and reduce systemic perfusion; conversely, large doses of induction agent may reduce SVR so much that shunt flow is reversed causing reduced PBF, worsened shunt, and desaturation. Propofol profoundly decreases SVR and MAP, which alters shunt dynamics to favour right to left flow and cyanosis. Hyperventilation reduces PVR by removing CO_2 and phenylephrine increases SVR, favouring a left to right shunt, improving pulmonary blood flow and reducing cyanosis. PEEP increases PVR.

Peyton JM, White MC. Anaesthesia for correction of congenital heart disease (for the specialist or senior trainee). *Continuing Education in Anaesthesia Critical Care & Pain* 2012; 12 (1): 23–27.

White MC, Peyton JM. Anaesthetic management of children with congenital heart disease for non-cardiac surgery. *Continuing Education in Anaesthesia Critical Care & Pain* 2012; 12 (1): 17–22.

10. D

Dilated cardiomyopathy results in impaired ventricular function secondary to progressive dilatation. Patients present with symptoms of chronic heart failure, embolic events, or arrhythmias. The important anaesthetic management aims are to maintain sinus rhythm, avoid tachycardia, and reduce or avoid increases in afterload. Cautious fluid management is important and should be goal directed. Preload should be maintained especially in the presence of elevated left ventricular end diastolic pressure, but fluid overload should be avoided.

Davies MR, Cousins J. Cardiomyopathy and anaesthesia. *Continuing Education in Anaesthesia Critical Care & Pain,* 2009; 9 (6): 189–193.

11. E

Pacemakers are coded as per a standard international system.

The first letter denotes chamber paced (V, ventricle; A, atrium; D, dual).

The second is chamber sensed (V, A, D)

The third is the mode of response (T, triggered; I, inhibited; D, dual).

The fourth letter denotes any programmable functions.

The fifth letter refers to special antitachycardia factors.

Diprose P, Pierce T. Anaesthesia for patients with pacemakers and similar devices. *Continuing Education in Anaesthesia, Critical Care & Pain* 2001; 1 (6): 166–170.

12. A

A preoperative FEV_1 of ≥1.5 L generally indicates suitability for lobectomy. Less than this would require further investigation and may preclude surgery.

If qualitative lung function tests confirm a predicted postoperative FEV_1 ≥40% and a predicted postoperative TLCO ≥40%, it would be safe to proceed to surgery.

Arterial $PaCO_2$ ≥6 kPa does not appear to be an independent predictor of poor outcome.

Oxygen saturation ≤90% has been associated with an increased risk of complications.

Gould G, Pearce A. Assessment of suitability for lung resection. *Continuing Education in Anaesthesia Critical Care & Pain* 2006; 6 (3): 97–100.

13. A

The transplanted heart has no autonomic innervation and the resting heart rate will sit around 100 bpm due to loss of vagal tone. This denervation also alters the pharmacological response to some commonly used anaesthetic drugs.

Vagolytics such as atropine and glycopyrrolate have no effect on a denervated heart.

Metaraminol would not treat the bradycardia.

Ephedrine, adrenaline (epinephrine), and isoprenaline could all be used to give positive chronotropy but they should be used cautiously as there may be an exaggerated response. Adenosine also demonstrates denervation hypersensivity and should be used in smaller doses.

Morgan-Hughes N, Hood G. Anaesthesia for the patient with a cardiac transplant *Continuing Education in Anaesthesia, Critical Care & Pain* 2002; 2 (3): 74–78.

14. B

Wherever possible, use should be made of synergistic, balanced, multimodal analgesia. Thoracotomy is notoriously painful postoperatively and creates a challenging acute postoperative pain management issue. Additionally, good acute pain management in thoracotomy may reduce the incidence of chronic neuropathic pain. The decision as to which technique to use for a particular patient is usually a matter of the anaesthetist's preference and local unit practices. Regional and neuraxial methods have obvious advantages but are associated with patchy coverage and a significant failure rate. Some afferent routes will not be blocked by the techniques described above (for example diaphragmatic irritation via the phrenic nerve) and many patients will also have chest drains inserted. If additional systemic analgesics can be administered, global analgesia will be improved. Regular paracetamol, NSAIDs where appropriate, parenteral or oral opioids are good choices in addition to a regional technique, embracing the doctrine of balanced multimodal analgesia.

Hughes R, Gao F. Pain control for thoracotomy. *Continuing Education in Anaesthesia, Critical Care & Pain* 2005; 5 (2): 56–60.

15. B

EURO Score is a commonly used worldwide risk stratification for patients undergoing cardiac surgery. It scores patient-, cardiac-, and operation-related factors to predict operative mortality. All answers are scored but an ejection fraction of <20% conveys the biggest score and therefore conveys the greatest risk.

EuroScore. The official website of the euroSCORE cardiac surgery scoring system. Available at: http://www.euroscore.org

16. D

The patient has not given informed consent; there has been no discussion about the risks and benefits for either an epidural or a paravertebral block, therefore these are not appropriate, especially at ST3/4 stage.

The patient does not necessarily require to be kept asleep in ICU.

PCA morphine would be an acceptable and safe method of providing analgesia.

Association of Anaesthetists of Great Britain and Ireland. AAGBI: Consent for anaesthesia 2017. *Anaesthesia* 2017; **72**: 93–105.

Dennehy L, White S. Consent, assent, and the importance of risk stratification. *British Journal of Anaesthesia* 2012; 109, (1): 40–46.

Hughes R, Gao F. Pain control for thoracotomy. *Continuing Education in Anaesthesia, Critical Care & Pain* 2005; 5 (2): 56–60.

17. D

A left-sided double lumen tube should be avoided as the staple line for pneumonectomy will be across the tube position. The same applies to using a bronchial blocker. All the others are possible but right sided is the best choice as it provides ready ability to isolate/suction as necessary.

Ng A, Swanevelder J. Hypoxaemia during one-lung anaesthesia. *Continuing Education in Anaesthesia Critical Care & Pain* 2010; 10 (4): 117–122.

18. D

The patient can be assumed to have a secondary spontaneous pneumothorax due to his age >50 years and significant smoking history. However, the pneumothorax is small based on the chest X-ray measurement and there are no obvious signs of current respiratory compromise. Therefore, an initial attempt can be made at aspirating air with a 16–18G cannula. The volume should be less than 2.5 L and the attempt at aspiration should abruptly cease indicating an expanded lung with no ongoing air leaks. A follow-up chest X-ray should demonstrate an improvement in pneumothorax size (<1 cm), otherwise a chest drain will subsequently be required.

If a secondary pneumothorax is larger (>2 cm) or the patient is breathless, then chest drain insertion is the correct initial action. All patients with a secondary pneumothorax should be admitted, commenced on oxygen therapy, and observed for 24 hours.

BTS Pleural Disease Guideline. British Thoracic Society Pleural Disease Guideline Group: A sub-group of the British Thoracic Society Standards of Care Committee. British Thoracic Society. Available at: https://www.brit-thoracic.org.uk/standards-of-care/guidelines/bts-pleural-disease-guideline/

19. D

Changes in airway pressures occur commonly during thoracic procedures. The clue as to their cause is often related to the most recent intervention. This should be considered as well as general differential diagnoses. In this case the patient has just been turned onto their side and even slight movement of the endotracheal tube can change airway pressures significantly if, for example, the tube moves further into a main bronchus or occludes a lobar bronchus. Positioning of the tube should be reconfirmed each time the patient position is changed.

Auscultation of the chest may reveal areas without air entry or reduced air entry but this is less reliable due to transmitted sounds and ambient noise in theatre.

If the patient is thought to be coughing, then suctioning of mucous and ensuring adequate muscle relaxation would be relevant.

The capnography trace may confirm an obstructive pattern of air flow but may also be normal. It does not help to identify the cause of the problem.

Anaesthesia UK. Double lumen endobronchial tubes updated. Updated 19/5/2010. Available at: http://www.frca.co.uk/article.aspx?articleid=246

20. A

The work of breathing is the work required to move the lungs both in inspiration and in expiration. During inspiration the work is to overcome airway resistance and during expiration it is to overcome compliance. On a pressure–volume curve the work of breathing is best indicated by the area within the hysteresis loop. Hysteresis means that the curves in inspiration and expiration are different.

In obstructive ventilation disorders such as asthma, more work is needed to overcome the flow resistance, particularly if positive intrapleural pressures are generated in expiration and this will be reflected in a larger hysteresis loop on the curve.

Grinnan DC, Truwit JD. Clinical review: Respiratory mechanics in spontaneous and assisted ventilation. *Critical Care* 2005; 9 (5): 472–484.

Anaesthesia UK. Physiology of ventilation. Updated 3/2/2010 http://www.frca.co.uk/article.aspx?article id=100423

1. **A patient requires posterior fossa surgery for excision of brain tumour in the sitting position. The best choice of monitor for detection of an intraoperative venous air embolism is:**
   A. Transoesophageal echocardiography
   B. Transoesophageal Doppler
   C. End-tidal CO_2
   C. Precordial stethoscope
   D. Precordial Doppler

2. **A 23-year-old man with complete transection of his spinal cord at T1 following an accident five months ago presents for a cystoscopy and urethral dilatation. He is known to have muscle spasms and has had one previous episode of autonomic dysreflexia. His body mass index (BMI) is 38. Which of the following would be the most appropriate anaesthetic technique?**
   A. No anaesthesia is required
   B. Lumbar epidural
   C. Low-dose spinal
   D. General anaesthesia with LMA
   E. Sedation with midazolam

3. **A 24-year-old man presents to the emergency department following a fall with a head injury. There are no obvious extracranial injuries. His Glasgow Coma Scale (GCS) is 6/15. You intubate him with manual in-line stabilization of his cervical spine. What is the most important management step to prevent secondary injury?**
   A. Maintain a mean arterial pressure (MAP) >80–90 mmHg
   B. Maintain a $PaCO_2$ of 4.0–4.5 kPA
   C. Aim for a blood glucose of 6–10 mmol
   D. Actively cool the patient to 35°C
   E. Maintain a PaO_2 >20 kPA

4. **A 26-year-old female presents with subarachnoid haemorrhage (SAH). She has no significant past medical history. On your arrival her eyes are open spontaneously, speech is confused, and she is localizing to pain on the right side only. Pupils are equal and reactive. What is the most appropriate clinical severity grade attributed?**
    A. Grade 1
    B. Grade 2
    C. Grade 3
    D. Grade 4
    E. Grade 5

5. **You are anaesthetizing a patient who is receiving posterior fossa surgery in the prone position. Their head is in a three-pin clamp. There is a sudden cardiovascular collapse proceeding immediately to cardiac arrest. The correct sequence of actions is:**
    A. Remain prone, clamp remains, commence posterior compressions
    B. Remain prone, commence posterior compressions, release head from clamp
    C. Remain prone, release head from clamp, commence posterior compressions
    D. Release head clamp, leave pins *in situ*, turn supine and commence compressions
    E. Remove all pins, turn patient supine, commence compressions

6. **You are taking a 64-year-old man with learning difficulties for magnetic resonance imaging (MRI) of the brain under anaesthesia. The presence of which of the following would be a contraindication to this procedure?**
    A. Prosthetic hip replacement
    B. Sternotomy wires for previous coronary artery bypass graft (CABG)
    C. Cochlear implant
    D. Plate in wrist from previous open reduction and internal fixation (ORIF)
    E. Metal heart valve

7. **A 28-year-old man has complete transection of this spinal cord at T4 following a road traffic accident 18 months ago. He is coming to theatre for insertion of a Baclofen pump. In theatre reception he complains of headache and flushing and his blood pressure is 194/98 mmHg. What would be the most appropriate initial step?**
    A. Re-check blood pressure
    B. Perform an ECG
    C. Exclude bladder obstruction
    D. Give diazepam pre-medication
    E. Take blood cultures

8. **A 37-year-old woman suffered a SAH four days ago. She is a smoker with no past medical history of note. The aneurysm was secured with coiling. Her GCS is currently 15 and there is no neurological deficit. The most common cause of a delayed neurological deficit now is:**

   A. Delayed cerebral ischaemia

   B. Hydrocephalus

   C. Seizure

   D. Re-bleeding

   E. Cerebral oedema

9. **A 42-year-old man presents for transphenoidal excision of pituitary adenoma. He originally presented with refractory hypertension, diabetes, and central obesity. The most likely endocrine abnormality is:**

   A. Hyperprolactinaemia

   B. Antidiuretic hormone (ADH) hyposecretion

   C. Thyroid stimulating hormone (TSH) hypersecretion

   D. Adrenocorticotropic hormone (ACTH) hypersecretion

   E. Growth hormone hypersecretion

10. **You assess a 46-year-old woman for percutaneous endoscopic gastrostomy (PEG) tube insertion. She has a six-month progressive neurological condition with chorea, dystonia, and pyramidal signs. She is suspected to have variant Creutzfeldt–Jakob disease. The most appropriate advice is:**

    A. No risk from routine contact, no isolation, disposable airway equipment, disposable surgical endoscope

    B. No risk from routine contact, no isolation, disposable airway equipment, reusable surgical endoscope

    C. Barrier nursing, isolation, disposable airway equipment, disposable surgical endoscope

    D. Barrier nursing, isolation, disposable airway equipment, reusable surgical endoscope

    E. No risk from routine contact, no isolation, reusable airway equipment, reusable surgical endoscope

11. **A 72-year-old woman with a one-year history of myasthenia gravis presents for wide local excision of breast cancer. She has no other significant past medical history. Her medication includes Pyridostigmine 90 mg three times per day. Preoperative investigation revealed a forced vital capacity (FVC) of 4.2 L, and normal echocardiography and ECG. She is of average height and normal BMI. She is able to manage one flight of stairs. She has no swallowing problems. There is no ITU bed currently available. What is the best plan?**

   A. Postpone surgery until ITU bed availability
   B. Proceed with spontaneous breathing technique on laryngeal mask airway (LMA), High Dependency Unit (HDU) postoperatively
   C. Intubate with an opiate based technique avoiding muscle relaxants, HDU postoperatively
   D. Give suxamethonium, intubate, HDU postoperatively
   E. Give non-depolarizing muscle relaxant, intubate, HDU postoperatively

12. **Which of the following operative positions is best avoided in routine posterior fossa neurosurgery?**

   A. Trendelenburg
   B. Supine
   C. Prone
   D. Park bench
   E. Lateral

13. **A 22-year-old man has suffered a diffuse axonal injury following car crash. He has spinal immobilization in place in ITU. GCS is 6 despite removal of sedation. Spinal fixation is *in situ*. What is the most appropriate course of action regarding spinal immobilization?**

   A. Computerized tomography (CT) neck, remove collar if normal
   B. CT neck, collar remains if normal
   C. Await improvement in GCS
   D. MRI neck, remove collar if normal
   E. MRI neck, collar remains if normal

14. **You anaesthetize a patient with well controlled epilepsy for elective inguinal hernia repair. They had taken their usual antiepileptic medication while fasting. In recovery they have a self-terminating tonic–clonic seizure. The correct advice is:**

   A. Driving not affected
   B. No driving for at least three months
   C. No driving for at least six months
   D. No driving for at least nine months
   E. No driving for at least 12 months

15. **You are asked to provide an anaesthetic opinion for a patient being considered for awake craniotomy. Which of the following is an absolute contraindication for awake craniotomy?**
    A. Obstructive sleep apnoea
    B. Learning difficulties
    C. Patient anxiety
    D. Language barrier
    E. Inability to lie still

16. **EEG-based depth of anaesthesia monitors have been used in an attempt to reduce awareness during general anaesthesia. Depth of anaesthesia monitoring should be used:**
    A. When thiopental is used as the induction agent for general anaesthesia
    B. During general anaesthesia for cardiac surgery
    C. During total intravenous anaesthesia (TIVA) with neuromuscular block
    D. During caesarean section under general anaesthesia
    E. During all general anaesthesia

17. **A patient is undergoing posterior fossa surgery for an acoustic neuroma. The anaesthetic induction was uneventful and the patient is haemodynamically stable. Half an hour into the operation, you notice a sudden reduction in end-tidal CO_2 waveform with a drop in blood pressure from 115/65 mmHg to 78/42 mmHg. What is the most immediate action to take next?**
    A. Aspirate air from the central venous catheter
    B. Administer metaraminol bolus
    C. Ask the surgeon to flood the operative field with fluid
    D. Increase FiO_2 to 1.0
    E. Give adrenaline (epinephrine) 0.1 mg IV bolus

18. **A 42-year-old woman presents to the Emergency Department complaining of new onset pins and needles in both legs. They are not painful but she feels they are becoming weak. On examination, power is 4/5 bilaterally and the patellar and Achilles tendon reflexes are absent. Lower limb pulses are present and normal. Colour is normal with no muscle wasting or skin changes. What is the most likely diagnosis?**
    A. Diabetic neuropathy
    B. Vascular insufficiency
    C. Multiple sclerosis
    D. Guillain–Barré syndrome
    E. Myasthenia gravis

19. **A 47-year-old woman is referred to the pain clinic by the neurosurgeons. She has low back pain and radiating down to her ankle on the left. MRI scan shows bulging discs at L4,5 and L5,S1. She is reluctant to proceed with surgical options at present. What is the best option to facilitate non-surgical management of this patient?**

    A. Regular acupuncture
    B. Caudal epidural steroid injections
    C. Facet joint injections
    D. Titrate opioid analgesia as required
    E. Refer to pain management programme

20. **A 37-year-old man is admitted to ITU following a high-speed road traffic accident. He has undergone an emergency laparotomy for liver laceration. A postoperative CT scan of his head showed a possible small haematoma. In ITU his renal function is deteriorating and his platelet count is falling. You are called to urgently review him when the nurse notices his right pupil to be newly fixed and dilated when performing neuro observations. What is the most appropriate action to take next?**

    A. Arrange an urgent repeat CT head
    B. Arrange transfer to the nearest neurosurgical unit
    C. Speak to haematology about giving pooled platelets
    D. Insert an arterial line
    E. Prescribe intravenous mannitol 0.5 g/kg

1. E

Precordial Doppler is the most sensitive non-invasive monitor, simple and able to detect as little as 0.015 mL/kg/min of intracardiac air. Precordial stethoscope requires a large amount of air to be entrained before detection of the classic millwheel murmur. End-tidal CO_2 is not specific to air embolism. Transoesophageal monitors are more sensitive than precordial Doppler but are invasive, expensive, and can be associated with complications such as oesophageal injury.

Jagannathan S, Krovvidi H. Anaesthetic considerations for posterior fossa surgery. *Continuing Education in Anaesthesia Critical Care & Pain* 2014; 14 (5): 202–206.

2. C

If site of surgery is below the level of the lesion and is complete no anaesthesia may be required unless the patient suffers from muscle spasms or autonomic dysreflexia (ADR). That is therefore not appropriate in this case.

Spinal anaesthesia is safe and is an effective way to abolish muscle spasms and ADR.

Epidurals may be unreliable for general or urological procedures.

Sedation does not reliably abolish muscle spasms or ADR.

A general anaesthetic would be an acceptable technique but intubation would be preferable as this patient has a high thoracic lesion and would have paralysis of his intercostal and abdominal wall muscles. He would be prone to hypoventilation and have reduced lung compliance. He would also be more at risk of aspiration as he has a high BMI and slower gastric emptying.

Petsas A, Drake J. Perioperative management for patients with a chronic spinal cord injury. *Continuing Education in Anaesthesia Critical Care & Pain* 2015; 15 (3): 123–130.

3. A

The main targets to avoid secondary brain injury are intubation and ventilation of anyone with a GCS <8. Then aim for PaO_2 >13 kPa, $PaCO_2$ 4.5–5 kPa, a MAP >80–90 mmHg, and normoglycaemia. Hyperthermia should also be avoided.

The most important of these are blood pressure control and maintaining oxygenation.

Episodes of hypotension or hypoxia are associated with a poorer outcome.

Dinsmore J. Traumatic brain injury: an evidence-based review of management. *Continuing Education in Anaesthesia Critical Care & Pain* 2013; 13 (6): 189–195.

4. C

There are more than 40 grading systems that can be used to describe the severity of SAH. A frequently used scale based on clinical signs is the World Federation of Neurosurgeons Scale

(WFNS) and is graded 1–5 based on GCS and motor deficit. It is related to prognosis. This patient has a GCS of E4, M5, V4 (total 13/15) with a hemiparetic motor deficit evident.

Clinically based scales are subject to interprofessional variability on assessment but do provide a means of summarized communication between team members and the regional neurological centre (Table 9.1).

Table 9.1 Severity of SAH grading

Grade	WFNS description
1	GCS 15, no motor deficit
2	GCS 13–14, no motor deficit
3	GCS 13–14 with motor deficit
4	GCS 7–12, with or without motor deficit
5	GCS 3–6, with or without motor deficit

Reprinted by permission from Springer, *Neurocritical Care*, 2, 2, Rosen DS, MacDonald RL, Subarachnoid hemorrhage grading scales, pp. 110–118. Copyright © 2005, Humana Press Inc.

Rosen DS, Macdonald RL. SAH grading scales: a systematic review. *Neurocritical Care* 2005; 1: 110–118.

Luoma A, Reddy U. Acute management of aneurysmal subarachnoid haemorrhage. *Continuing Education in Anaesthesia Critical Care & Pain* 2013; 13 (2): 52–58.

5. B

Cardiopulmonary resuscitation (CPR) should not be delayed and there is no immediate need to turn the patient to the supine position; CPR should be started with the patient in the prone position. The head can be released from the clamp on the operating table rather than trying to release the head from the pins. This reduces the risk of injuring the scalp, leaving a bleeding pin-hole, or the operator being injured by the pins. The surgeon can support the patient's head while CPR is administered.

Working Group of the Resuscitation Council (UK), Neuroanaesthesia Society of Great Britain and Ireland and Society of British Neurological Surgeons. Management of cardiac arrest during neurosurgery in adults—Guidelines for healthcare providers. Resuscitation Council UK 2014. Available at: https://www.google.com/url?sa=t&rct=j&q=&esrc=s&source=web&cd=1&cad=rja&uact=8&ved=2ahUKEwi5juzd9LDfAhX9QhUIHbsKAv8QFjAAegQIChAC&url=http%3A%2F%2Fwww.resus.org.uk%2FEasysiteWeb%2Fgetresource.axd%3FAssetID%3D870%26type%3DFull%26servicetype%3DAttachment&usg=AOvVaw1evUoWDJeM2-IrB3s82mpb

6. C

Absolute contraindications to MRI include cochlear implants, intra-ocular foreign bodies, and ferromagnetic neurovascular clips. Cardiac pacemakers and implantable defibrillators would also be contraindicated as these may malfunction within the 5 Gauss line.

Most modern prosthesis are non-ferromagnetic. General surgical clips, artificial heart valves, and sternal wires are usually deemed safe as they are fixed in place by fibrous tissue.

Stuart G. Understanding magnetic resonance imaging. Anaesthesia Tutorial of the Week 177. Available at: http://www.frca.co.uk/Documents/177%20Understanding%20Magnetic%20resonance%20imaging.pdf

7. C

This is describing autonomic dysreflexia and the most important first step is to exclude urinary obstruction before administration of drugs.

Petsas A, Drake J. Perioperative management for patients with a chronic spinal cord injury. *Continuing Education in Anaesthesia Critical Care & Pain* 2015; 15 (3) 123–130.

8. A

Those with poor clinical grade SAH and/or large amounts of subarachnoid and intraventricular blood are at particularly high risk of complications.

The risk of re-bleeding is greatest immediately after the initial haemorrhage, with rates of 5–10% within the first three days. Twenty to 30% of patients develop hydrocephalus, usually within the first three days but it may also be delayed. Clinical seizures are uncommon, occurring in only 1–7% of patients. In patients with an unsecured aneurysm, they are often a sign of a re-bleed. Although seizures should be treated aggressively, the use of prophylactic anticonvulsants is associated with a worse outcome after SAH and is not recommended.

Delayed cerebral ischaemia occurs in >60% with the greatest risk between days 4 and 10 and may even occur in the absence of vasospasm. Smokers are particularly at risk for vasospasm. This patient is a smoker starting at day 4 post bleed.

Luoma A, Reddy U. Acute management of aneurysmal subarachnoid haemorrhage. *Continuing Education in Anaesthesia Critical Care & Pain* 2013; 13 (2): 52–58.

9. D

This patient presents with features of Cushing's disease. This is an excess of glucocorticoid due to hypersecretion of ACTH from a pituitary corticotrophin adenoma, the term *Cushing's syndrome* being applied to a non-specific state of chronic glucocorticoid excess regardless of cause. Surgical excision is the definitive management, but medical treatment may reverse much of the effects of excess glucocorticoid and considerably reduces perioperative risk. The typical habitus of Cushing's syndrome is one of truncal obesity, moon face and thin extremities. Glucose intolerance is seen in almost two-thirds of patients with Cushing's disease, half of whom will have frank diabetes.

Menon R, Murphy P, Lindley A. Anaesthesia and pituitary disease. *Continuing Education in Anaesthesia Critical Care & Pain* 2011; 11 (4): 133–137.

10. A

Abnormal prion protein is not completely removed by conventional sterilization methods, including autoclaving. This poses problems for transmission of prion disease by contaminated surgical equipment. This is relevant when a patient with CJD, or at increased risk of CJD, has a procedure involving tissue which is deemed of medium or high risk.

With the advent of CJD, there has been a need for airway equipment to become single use. In most centres, disposable laryngoscope blades and single-use laryngeal masks are now in routine use. While fibreoptic intubating endoscopes have until recently been sterilized and reused, disposable endoscopes are now available. Anaesthetizing a patient with suspected CJD is essentially similar to routine practice with no particular barrier measures, routine contact infection risk, or isolation required. In this case, the gastrointestinal lymphoid tissue is of medium infectivity risk so the surgical scope should be incinerated.

Porter M-C, Leemans M. Creutzfeldt–Jakob disease. *Continuing Education in Anaesthesia Critical Care & Pain* 2013; 13 (4): 119–124.

11. B

She has grade 2a myasthenia gravis—mild, generalized, responding to therapy. She has a low risk of requiring prolonged ventilation postoperatively as myasthenia gravis history is less than six years, no concurrent respiratory disease, pyridostigmine <750 mg/day, and FVC >2.9 L. HDU postoperatively is appropriate. She is having a short peripheral site procedure and appears suitable for LMA as no swallowing problems and normal BMI. This technique also avoids the use of ventilation and muscle relaxants (reduced effect of DMR and increased effect of NDMR).

Banerjee A. Anaesthesia and myasthenia gravis. Anaesthesia Tutorial of the Week 122. Available at: http://www.frca.co.uk/Documents/122%20Myasthenia%20Gravis.pdf

Thavasothy M, Hirsch N. Myasthenia gravis. *BJA CEPD Reviews* 2002; 2 (3): 88–90.

12. A

Posterior fossa surgery is commonly performed in supine, prone, sitting, lateral, and park bench positions. The Trendelenburg position would lead to increased venous engorgement although may be used in an emergency, when air embolism is suspected, to place the surgical field below the level of the heart. Park bench position is a modification of the lateral position where the patient is positioned semi-prone with the head flexed and facing the floor. This facilitates greater access to midline structures and, in selected patients, avoids the need for the prone position.

Jagannathan S, Krovvidi H. Anaesthetic considerations for posterior fossa surgery. *Continuing Education in Anaesthesia Critical Care & Pain* 2014; 14 (5): 202–206.

13. A

The question describes a patient with a poor prognosis who is likely to remain low GCS for an unknown period of time. 'Clearing' the cervical spine requires an awake cooperative patient. However prolonged, unnecessary spinal immobilization also represents significant risks to the patient. Clinicians must decide what investigation, or combination of investigations, provides them with enough evidence to either diagnose a cervical spine injury or exclude it. MRI in the trauma ICU patient presents monitoring/transfer/access difficulties.

High-resolution CT should provide satisfactory images with 3D reconstruction. If these images are reported as normal, by an experienced radiologist, then the risk of the patient having a significant, missed injury is small enough to warrant safe removal of spinal immobilization.

Harrison P, Cairns C. Clearing the cervical spine in the unconscious patient. *Continuing Education in Anaesthesia Critical Care & Pain* 2008; 8 (4): 117–120.

14. E

No driving for 12 months.

If seizures have occurred while awake and conscious the driving licence is taken away for at least 12 months. The patient can reapply if they have been seizure free following this time.

If the seizure occurred because a doctor changed or reduced the anti-epilepsy medicine, they can reapply after six months free of seizures. If the patient has a bus/coach/lorry license the rules are much stricter with five years seizure free required.

Epilepsy and driving. Available at: https://www.gov.uk/epilepsy-and-driving

15. E

A patient who is unable to lie still for the duration of the operation is an absolute contraindication for awake craniotomy. Clearly this may be due to a variety of causes—physical or psychological. All the other answers are relative contraindications.

Awake craniotomy is an important technique for increased lesion removal and minimizing damage to eloquent cortex. An important aspect of an awake craniotomy is the patient selection and preparation by the multidisciplinary team. The patient must know what to expect and the anaesthetic risks involved.

Burnand C, Sebastian J. Anaesthesia for awake craniotomy, *Continuing Education in Anaesthesia Critical Care & Pain*. 2014; 14 (1): 6–11.

16. C

Depth of anaesthesia monitoring is recommended during TIVA. The other answers include risk factors for awareness.

Association of Anaesthetists of Great Britain and Ireland. Recommendations for standards of monitoring during anaesthesia and recovery 2015. *Anaesthesia* 2016; 71: 85–93.

17. C

The most likely cause of this scenario is air embolism due to an open vessel in the surgical field therefore flooding the site with saline will prevent further in-drawing of air.

Air embolism is a rare but serious consequence of intracranial surgery. During acoustic neuroma surgery it can happen if the sigmoid sinus or jugular venous sinus are breached. The patient is usually head up for this procedure and air intake is minimized by having the surgeon immediately flood the surgical field, cover it, and tilt the patient head down.

Increasing the FiO_2 (D), and using vasopressors (B and E) are supportive measures which may also be required. Aspirating air from the CVP line (A) is impractical, unlikely to be effective, and risks exposing the circulation to further air.

Auscultation of the chest typically reveals a mill wheel murmur which helps confirm the diagnosis.

Webber S, Andrzejowski J, Francis G. Gas embolism in anaesthesia. *BJA CEPD Reviews*, 2002; 2 (2): 53–57.

18. D

Guillain–Barré disease is an ascending symmetrical polyneuropathy affecting somatic and autonomic nerves. It is characterized by motor weakness but sensory changes also occur.

A and B would be painful conditions with normal power and associated skin changes such as ulceration or venous congestion.

Motor neurone disease has no sensory component.

Multiple sclerosis affects random areas of the body and is not symmetrical.

Myasthenia gravis has brisk tendon reflexes and weakness characterized by fatigability.

Fokke C, van den Berg B, Drenthen J, et al. Diagnosis of Guillain–Barré syndrome and validation of Brighton criteria. *Brain* 2014; 137 (1): 33–43.

19. E

Self-management is the key to long-term success in pain management, giving the patient an internal locus of control, tools, information, and support to deal with chronic pain and flare ups. Long-term management will require pacing, setting objectives, and practising mindfulness or relaxation.

Regular acupuncture works for some patients but is not a long-term solution nor is it recommended for low back pain (NICE CG59). Caudal steroid injections will help the pain but only in the short term. It is not practical to repeat these at frequent intervals. Facet joint injections will not help the pain which is most likely due to disc impingement or compression of nerves or disc pathology causing inflammation around nerve roots.

Opioids are not recommended as a long-term solution in back pain. They can be used with care, for short periods with defined objectives agreed with patient.

Low back pain and sciatica in over 16s: assessment and management NICE guideline [NG59]. Available at: https://www.nice.org.uk/guidance/ng59

20. E.

A unilateral fixed dilated pupil after head injury indicates imminent herniation and must be decompressed immediately. This can be achieved with a bolus dose of mannitol 0.5 g/kg.

Mannitol is an osmotic diuretic which draws fluid from neurons reducing intracranial volume and pressure for a short period to allow preparation for urgent craniotomy.

The acute problem is not due to a bleeding diathesis so treatment with clotting products is not appropriate.

There is no time to repeat the CT of head. The diagnosis of raised intracranial pressure is a clinical one in this scenario. Likewise, inserting an arterial line may be useful but will not prevent deterioration of the patient's clinical condition.

Control of intracranial hypertension. Available at: http://www.trauma.org/archive/neuro/icpcontrol.html

1. You assess a two-day-old baby requiring surgery for testicular torsion. The baby was born at 39 weeks' gestation after an uneventful pregnancy and delivery. The baby is of average weight. What is the correct does of intravenous paracetamol?
   A. 3.5 mg
   B. 10 mg
   C. 15 mg
   D. 26 mg
   E. 53 mg

2. You anaesthetize a four-year-old child for exploration of groin. He has no relevant past medical history and has not had a general anaesthetic (GA) before. After IV induction you insert a size 2 LMA and he is spontaneously breathing oxygen/air/sevoflurane on an Ayre's T piece. You give 2 mg of morphine IV. After 30 min into the operation you note a rising $FiCO_2$. All other parameters are within normal range. The most likely cause is:
   A. Hypoventilation secondary to opioid
   B. Malignant hyperpyrexia
   C. Soda lime exhausted
   D. Fresh gas flow too low
   E. Fresh gas flow too high

3. You anaesthetize a seven-year-old boy for manipulation of forearm fracture. On attaching the electrocardiogram (ECG) you notice multiple round bruises of different ages all over his torso. You are concerned the child may have suffered non-accidental injury. It is 10 pm. The best action you should take is:
   A. Notify your Consultant
   B. Phone the on-call social worker
   C. Phone the police
   D. Phone the court
   E. Notify the hospital-designated child protection doctor

4. **You perform an inguinal nerve block on a seven-year-old child for operative management of undescended testis on the same side. The safest way to avoid inadvertent intravascular injection is:**
   A. Monitor closely with ECG, non-invasive blood pressure (NIBP), and pulse oximetry
   B. Using local anaesthetic with adrenaline (epinephrine)
   C. Regular aspiration during injection
   D. Using a nerve stimulator to guide placement
   E. Observing the maximum safe dosage as per the child's weight

5. **Lidocaine 2% spray to the vocal cords may reduce the incidence of laryngospasm following tonsillectomy. Which best describes the pharmacodynamics of this?**
   A. It blocks the recurrent laryngeal nerves bilaterally
   B. It blocks sympathetic efferents
   C. It blocks parasympathetic afferents
   D. It paralyses the smooth muscle of the larynx
   E. It blocks superior recurrent laryngeal nerve

6. **A ten-month-old infant presents for elective herniotomies under GA. He appears well though routine examination reveals a soft systolic murmur; the rest of the examination is normal. The most appropriate action to take is:**
   A. Postpone surgery and obtain an urgent cardiac echocardiogram
   B. Postpone surgery and refer the child cardiologist for investigation
   C. Assume this is an innocent murmur and proceed
   D. Proceed with anaesthesia giving antibiotic cover
   E. Proceed with surgery under local anaesthesia

7. **You are in a restaurant when a mother frantically calls for assistance with her three-year-old daughter who appears to be choking. The child is conscious, and appears to be coughing but no noise is made. What is the most appropriate immediate action?**
   A. Continue to encourage coughing
   B. Deliver five back blows
   C. Call for help (999) and deliver five abdominal thrusts
   D. Perform a finger sweep under direct vision to dislodge the object
   E. Place the child in the recovery position

8. **You anaesthetize a 6-year-old child for adenotonsillectomy. After the Boyle–Davis gag has been positioned, you notice the patient's abdomen moving excessively. You diagnose partial airway obstruction, confirmed by capnography. What is most likely to be the cause of this?**
   A. The LMA has moved
   B. The LMA is too small
   C. The Boyle–Davis gag is too small
   D. The depth of anaesthesia is insufficient
   E. The child has aspirated gastric contents

9. **A nine-year-old boy with mild learning difficulties and an incarcerated inguinal hernia requires surgical repair. He is refusing medication and topical local anaesthetic. The parents are hyper-anxious. Which of the following is the most appropriate action?**
   A. Wait until child is calm before anaesthetizing him
   B. Restrain with parental consent and attempt gas induction
   C. Restrain with parental consent, give midazolam 0.5 mg/kg orally and wait 20 min
   D. Give IM ketamine 5 mg/kg and wait 5 min
   E. Restrain with parental consent and apply topical local anaesthetic cream to hands

10. **A three-year-old child has presented with coughing and mild stridor. The child is anaesthetized for investigation of the cause of these symptoms and a STORZ ventilating bronchoscope is inserted. What is the most correct statement regarding the use of a ventilating bronchoscope?**
    A. Oxygenation is usually maintained by jet ventilation
    B. It can only be used for diagnostic procedures
    C. Correctly sized scope for the child will allow an audible leak at a 20 cmH$_2$O pressure
    D. It is a fibreoptic scope
    E. No ventilation of the contralateral lung will occur if it is inserted endobronchially

11. **A five-year-old boy of African origin presents for an elective hernia surgery. His full blood count reveals his haemoglobin is 80 g/L. Which of the following is the best test to diagnose sickle cell disease?**
    A. Coagulation screen
    B. Sickledex test
    C. Reticulocyte count
    D. Haemoglobin electrophoresis
    E. Serum lactate dehydrogenase

12. **You review a two-year-old boy in the emergency department with difficulty breathing. He has had recent coryzal symptoms. No significant medical history. His breathing is noisy on inspiration with tracheal tug and accessory muscle use. His saturations are 94% on air, RR 40 breaths/min. His temperature is 37.5°C. The most likely diagnosis is:**

A. Epiglottitis

B. Bacterial tracheitis

C. Laryngomalacia

D. Croup

E. Asthma

13. **In the fetus, blood supplying the brain has a higher oxygen content than blood supplying the trunk and lower limbs. Which of the following statements is the best explanation for this?**

A. HbF has a higher oxygen affinity than adult haemoglobin

B. Metabolic autoregulation of the cerebral circulation

C. In the fetal circulation, blood with a higher oxygen content flows across the foramen ovale and into the carotid arteries via the left ventricle

D. The ductus arteriosus ensures that blood from the pulmonary artery bypasses the collapsed fetal lungs

E. The ductus venosus ensures that most oxygenated blood from the umbilical vein bypasses the portal circulation

14. **You attend the emergency department to review a six-year-old child with sudden onset breathing difficulty. On your arrival the child appears unwell with lip and tongue swelling, expiratory wheeze, and widespread erythematous rash. Saturations are 91% on oxygen. The child has no previous medical history. The most important drug treatment is:**

A. Chlorphenamine

B. Salbutamol

C. Hydrocortisone

D. Magnesium

E. Adrenaline (epinephrine)

15. **An eight-year-old boy requires circumcision under general anaesthesia. He is of normal weight and height for age. The best first choice of laryngeal mask size is:**

A. 1

B. 1½

C. 2

D. 2½

E. 3

16. **You review a four-year-old boy in the emergency department with difficulty breathing. He has no significant medical history. His breathing is noisy on inspiration with tracheal tug and accessory muscle use. He is sitting upright and drooling. His saturations are 92% on air, RR 60 breaths/min. His temperature is 39.3°C. The most appropriate immediate management is:**
    A. Nebulized budesonide
    B. IM dexamethasone
    C. Heliox
    D. Nebulized adrenaline (epinephrine)
    E. IM antibiotics

17. **You perform gas induction of anaesthesia in an uncooperative three-year-old child following failed attempt at IV cannulation. The child develops laryngospasm which does not resolve with simple measures. The fastest route to break laryngospasm in this child is:**
    A. Intravenous (IV) suxamethonium 1.5 mg/kg
    B. Intramuscular (IM) suxamethonium 3 mg/kg
    C. Intralingual (IL) suxamethonium 2 mg/kg
    D. Intramuscular suxamethonium 4 mg/kg
    E. Intraosseous (IO) suxamethonium 2 mg/kg

18. **A four-year-old child presents for circumcision. He has a runny nose, temperature of 37.2°C, chest is clear on auscultation, and is otherwise well. His father is particularly keen the child gets his operation today. You should:**
    A. Delay the operation two weeks until he is better
    B. Delay the operation six weeks until respiratory tract returns to normal
    C. Delay the operation to test for sickle cell anaemia
    D. Proceed with the operation using GA and caudal analgesia
    E. Proceed with the operation using GA and penile block analgesia

19. **A nine-year old child is fasting and requires maintenance fluid. They are of normal weight for age and have no history of significant fluid losses. What rate of maintenance intravenous fluid therapy would you estimate they require?**
    A. 66 mL/hour
    B. 104 mL/hour
    C. 78 mL/hour
    D. 260 mL/hour
    E. 90 mL/hour

20. **A eight-year-old girl requires emergency appendicectomy. She has normal height and weight for age. The best choice uncuffed endotracheal tube is:**

A. ID 5.0 mm tube, depth 16 cm at lips
B. ID 6.0 mm tube, depth 16 cm at lips
C. ID 5.5 mm tube, depth 14 cm at lips
D. ID 5.0 mm tube, depth 14 cm at lips
E. ID 6.0 mm tube, depth 16 cm at lips

1. D

An average neonate weighs approximately 3.5 kg. The paediatric dose of intravenous paracetamol is 15 mg/kg between 10 and 33 kg. However, according to MHRA guidance and the Safe Anaesthesia Liaison Group regarding neonates and children <10 kg, the dose is reduced to 7.5 mg/kg (3.5 kg × 7.5 mg/kg = 26.25 mg). This is because of increased risk of toxicity in the context of altered pharmacokinetics of developing organs.

Medicines and Healthcare Regulatory Agency. Intravenous paracetamol (Perfalgan): risk of accidental overdose. *Drug Safety Update* 2010; 3 (12): 2.

2. D

The question asks about rising fractional inspired CO_2. Answers A and B would cause a rise in the end tidal CO_2 only. The weight of a four-year-old child can be estimated at 17 or 18 kg.

The correct dose of morphine is 0.1–0.2 mg/kg so in this case an appropriate dose has been given.

Soda lime is not used with an Ayre's T piece.

The fresh gas flow (FGF) when using this breathing system must be at least two or three times the minute ventilation of the patient to prevent rebreathing and a rise of inspired CO_2. Having a gas flow that is higher than required is safe with no detrimental side effects for the patient but cost/waste/air pollution become relevant.

Harrison GA. Ayre's T-piece: a review of its modifications. *British Journal of Anaesthesia* 1964; 36: 115–120.

3. E

The anaesthetist has a duty of care to act upon any concerns they have regarding child safety and should ensure they are familiar with the local child protection policies within their organization.

Every organization has designated child protection doctors, nurses, and midwives with whom serious concerns can be raised and discussed either formally or informally. This is commonly the Consultant Paediatrician on call who can ensure the issue is managed by the child protection team if deemed necessary.

Good Medical Practice. Protecting children and young people. The responsibilities of all doctors. Available at: http://www.gmc-uk.org/guidance/ethical_guidance/13260.asp

Melarkode K, Wilkinson K. Child protection issues and the anaesthetist. *Continuing Education in Anaesthesia Critical Care & Pain* 2012; 12 (3): 123–127.

4. C

Note this is not a question about local anaesthetic toxicity, it is specifically about accidental intravascular injection, which is only one of the causes of local anaesthetic toxicity.

Regular aspiration during injection (answer C) is the only one which allows early detection of accidental intravascular injection. Monitoring as in option A would detect it but not avoid it; adrenaline (epinephrine) would increase the safe dosage and show a tachycardia but not protect against IV injection. D and E may prevent toxicity resulting from an excessive dose of local anaesthetic but not specifically due to intravenous injection.

AAGBI Safety Guideline. Management of severe local anaesthetic toxicity. Available at: https://www.aagbi.org/sites/default/files/la_toxicity_2010_0.pdf

Fisher QA, Shaffner DH, Yaster M. Detection of intravascular injection of regional anaesthetics in children. *Canadian Journal of Anesthesia* 1997; 44 (6): 592–598.

5. C

Laryngospasm occurs by contraction of the intrinsic muscles of the larynx, specifically the adductors. It is usually triggered by a peri-glottic stimulus mediated via the vagus nerve.

Lidocaine will block the afferent pathway to prevent the reflex efferent response of glottic closure.

The larynx is supplied by the superior laryngeal nerve above the vocal cords and the recurrent laryngeal nerve below the vocal cords. Both are branches of the vagal nerve and both would need to be blocked to prevent the efferent arc of the reflex.

Gavel G , Walker RWM. Laryngospasm in anaesthesia. *Continuing Education in Anaesthesia Critical Care & Pain*, 2014; 14 (2): 47–51.

Mihara T, Uchimoto K, Morita S, Goto T. The efficacy of lidocaine to prevent laryngospasm in children. A systematic review and meta-analysis. *Anaesthesia* 2014; 69 (12): 1388–1396.

6. B

The surgery is elective and non-urgent. Most murmurs are innocent murmurs, with less than 1% signifying congenital heart disease and most congenital heart disease is diagnosed before the age of three months. But, any child who is less than one year old should be thoroughly investigated by Paediatric Cardiologists as presentation may be slower and/or later.

Bhatia N, Barber N. Dilemmas in the preoperative assessment of children. *Continuing Education in Anaesthesia Critical Care & Pain* 2011; 11 (6): 214–218.

7. B

From the 2015 Paediatric BLS choking guidelines, if there is an ineffective cough in a conscious child (no noise, cannot vocalize, cyanosed) then five back blows should be immediately delivered followed by five abdominal thrusts (use chest thrusts in an infant to avoid solid organ damage). If the child were to become unconscious, the airway should be opened and anything visible could be removed, followed by commencing basic life support.

Resuscitation Council (UK). 2015 Paediatric choking. Available at: https://www.resus.org.uk/resuscitation-guidelines/paediatric-basic-life-support/#choking

8. A

The LMA is most likely to have moved: this is common during the move from anaesthetic room to theatre plus transfer of patient onto table. If not in the correct position the LMA will be obstructed when the Boyle–Davis gag is fully opened. Insertion of the gag is a time when vigilance is specifically required to confirm the airway remains patent post insertion.

An LMA which is too small should not cause obstruction in this way (although may not establish the best airway) and the Boyle–Davis gag used should the smallest possible to do the job.

Depth of anaesthesia can be reduced during transfer but should be confirmed as adequate before giving the surgeon permission to begin. Aspiration is less likely in a fasted child for an elective procedure.

Ravi R, Howell T. Anaesthesia for paediatric ear, nose, and throat surgery. *Continuing Education in Anaesthesia Critical Care & Pain* 2007; 7 (2): 33–37.

9. D

There is risk of surgical sequelae if he refuses to proceed.

The child is nine years old and older children will remember an unpleasant experience. This could persist into adulthood and the child may continue to be very anxious. Gas induction could prolong the experience and be difficult especially if regurgitation risk.

The dose of midazolam is usually 0.5 mg/kg and effect peaks at 20–30 min and then wears off. Timing is crucial. The child will probably spit out medicine and still require restraint and cannula.

This ketamine dose is correct for sedation. Duration of restraint is very brief to deliver IM injection and will work within 5 min effectively in 93–100% of children. Rapid action means the anaesthetist can observe effects and time cannulation for IV induction.

Topical LA will probably be peeled off, takes 30 min to work, and still need cooperation for cannula afterwards.

Tan L, Meakin GH. Anaesthesia for the uncooperative child. *Continuing Education in Anaesthesia Critical Care & Pain* 2010; 10 (2): 48–52.

10. C

Ventilation occurs by attaching a breathing system, usually the Jackson-Rees T- piece to its distal end. It can be used for diagnostic and therapeutic procedures. It is a rigid scope with an optical telescope sealing the distal end of the scope. Correct sizing allows a leak at a pressure of 20 cmH$_2$O. It has hole in its wall around 5 cm from the tip to allow ventilation of contralateral lung if inserted endobronchially.

Roberts S, Thornington RE. Paediatric bronchoscopy. *Continuing Education in Anaesthesia Critical Care & Pain* 2005; 5 (2): 41–44.

11. D

Haemoglobin electrophoresis is the definitive test. The Sickledex test can be useful in emergencies as it is a rapid easily performed bedside test. However, it only confirms the presence of HbS, it does not differentiate between the heterozygous (sickle cell trait) and the homozygous state (sickle cell disease).

Wilson M, Forsyth P, Whiteside J. Haemoglobinopathy and sickle cell disease. *Continuing Education in Anaesthesia Critical Care & Pain* 2010; 10 (1): 24–28.

12. D

This child has inspiratory stridor and is systemically fairly well with a mild pyrexia. Croup is a common cause of stridor in children of this age and is viral in origin. A classic sign is a seal-like barking cough. Epiglottitis is less common following *Haemophilus Influenza* B vaccination programmes and usually results in a child who is toxic/systemically unwell with prominent drooling and difficulty swallowing. It presents acutely in otherwise healthy children with a fever as high as 40°C. Epiglottic inflammation occurs quickly with the child sitting forward to use the accessory muscles of respiration and pain in the throat. Salivation is prominent with difficulty swallowing. Bacterial tracheitis is rare. Asthma would usually have a longer past history in an older child with expiratory obstruction. Laryngomalacia may also have a more chronic history and is rarer than croup in an otherwise well child (Table 10.1).

Table 10.1 Suggested factors in determining the diagnosis of croup versus epiglottitis

	Croup	Epiglottitis
Aetiology	Parainfluenza virus	*Haemophilus influenza*
Age	**4** months to 2 years	2–5 years
Onset	Subacute exacerbation of pre-existent URI	Acute
Temperature	Low-grade fever	High fever
Course	Usually mild, stridor may worsen at night	Rapid progress of symptoms
Symptoms	Barky cough, stridor	Dysphagia, sore throat, dysphonia, respiratory disease

Maloney E, Meakin GH. Acute stridor in children. *Continuing Education in Anaesthesia Critical Care & Pain* 2007; 7 (6): 183–186.

13. C

All the statements are true. However, only C answers the question directly. In D the ductus arteriosus enter the aorta distal to the branching to the carotids.

Murphy PJ. The fetal circulation. *Continuing Education in Anaesthesia Critical Care & Pain* 2005; 5 (4): 107–112.

Human Embryology. Online course for medical students. Module 16 Cardiovascular system. Embryo-fetal circulation and changes at birth. Available at: http://www.embryology.ch/anglais/pcardio/umstellung01.html

14. E

This patient has features of life-threatening anaphylaxis. The rash, swelling, and lack of medical history point away from pure asthma. The trigger is not clear from the history. All the medications can be used to treat anaphylaxis. Antihistamines are second-line drugs and unlikely to influence rapid recovery although their use is logical. Steroids will help shorten episodes and prevent further flares although will not have an immediate action. Magnesium is indicated in asthma—intravenous magnesium is a vasodilator and can cause hot flushes and make hypotension worse. Adrenaline (epinephrine) is the most important drug for the treatment of an anaphylactic reaction and should be given to all patients with life-threatening features. It works quickly to alter the course of the condition. As an alpha-receptor agonist, it reverses peripheral vasodilation and reduces oedema. Its beta-receptor agonist activity dilates the bronchial airways, increases the force of myocardial contraction, and suppresses histamine and leukotriene release. There are also beta-2 adrenergic receptors on mast cells that inhibit activation. Early adrenaline (epinephrine) reduces the severity of allergic reaction.

Emergency treatment of anaphylactic reactions, Guidelines for healthcare providers. Working Group of the Resuscitation Council (UK) January 2008. Resuscitation Council (UK). Available at: http://ww.resus.org.uk

15. D

Average weight may be estimated by Weight = (Age + 4) × 2 (1–10 years).

> LMA #1—<6.5 kg
> LMA #1.5—<13 kg

LMA #2—<20 kg
LMA #2.5—<25 kg
LMA #3—20–30 kg
LMA #4—> 30 kg

Emergency treatment of anaphylactic reactions: Guidelines for healthcare providers. Working Group of the Resuscitation Council (UK), January 2008. Available at: https://www.resus.org.uk/anaphylaxis/emergency-treatment-of-anaphylactic-reactions/

16. D

The clinical signs indicate an airway concern with elements of respiratory distress. This is most likely due to swelling in the upper airway probably of infective origin. Nebulized drugs are generally not distressing to a child presenting with an airway emergency. Parenteral administration could precipitate airway obstruction. Adrenaline (epinephrine) nebulized is likely to be effective quickly.

Maloney E, Meakin GH. Acute stridor in children. *Continuing Education in Anaesthesia Critical Care & Pain* 2007; 7 (6): 183–186.

17. C

The patient has no IV or IO access currently, which will require additional time to obtain and an extra pair of skilled hands. IL succinylcholine is essentially an IM injection into the body of the tongue. An IL injection of succinylcholine of 2 mg/kg has been studied in children. Full relaxation occurs in 75 seconds, and, therefore, relaxation of laryngospasm will be quicker than an IM injection in the skeletal muscles. Practically, IL succinylcholine requires injection directly into/around the airway which could potentially make an awkward airway even more difficult. While IL is the fastest onset route in this scenario, we suggest that most anaesthetists are likely to choose an IM injection (e.g. in deltoid) first in preference. The IM dose is 4 mg/kg (suggested maximum dose 200 mg).

Although the time taken for full paralysis is 3–4 min, the time taken to break laryngospasm will be 45 seconds to 1 min. Studies have shown that relaxation of the laryngeal muscles occurs before skeletal muscles and thus IM succinylcholine is a reasonable option.

Gavel G, Walker RWM. Laryngospasm in anaesthesia. *Continuing Education in Anaesthesia Critical Care & Pain* 2014; 14 (2): 47–51.

18. E

It is common for children to have runny noses and provided they are apyrexial and systemically well it is safe to proceed but it is important to provide excellent analgesia. For this operation the safest effective method would be by penile block with a GA.

You would not postpone to test for sickle cell. If there was a high index of suspicion you would carry on as if the child had sickle cell in the appropriate manner. You should keep them warm and well hydrated and avoid hypercarbia and hypoxia and tourniquets.

Shetty N, Sethi D. Paediatric anaesthesia for day surgery. Anaesthetic Tutorial of the Week 203. Available at: http://www.frca.co.uk/Documents/203%20Anaesthesia%20for%20paediatric%20day%20surgery.pdf

19. A

Estimated weight is (age + 4) × 2 = 26 kg assuming normality. Using the 4:2:1 regimen it works out as 66 mL/hour.

Wilson C. Paediatric Fluids. Anaesthesia UK. Available at: http://www.frca.co.uk/article.aspx?articleid=100481

20. E

Formulas based on age and height may fail to reliably predict the proper endotracheal tube (ETT) size in paediatric patients. Various equations are available although the individual patient should be considered in each case.

Predicted internal diameter tube size = age/4 + 4.5 is generally a better fit than age/4 + 4 up to 10 years, although both are often quoted. Therefore a 6.0-mm or 6.5-mm tube could be used in this patient, though only a 6.0 mm answer is offered as an option These formulas are typically applicable to children aged 1–12 years. Above age 12, typically most adult sizes (6.5–8.0) can be considered.

The Advanced Paediatric Life Support (APLS) guidelines recommend calculating tracheal tube insertion depth for children older than one year according to the formula: insertion depth (cm) for orotracheal intubation = age/2 + 12.

MacFarlane F. Paediatric anatomy and physiology and the basics of paediatric anaesthesia. World Anaesthesia Tutorial of the Week. Available at: https://www.aagbi.org/sites/default/files/7-Paediatric-anatomy-physiology-and-the-basics-of-paediatric-anaesthesia.pdf

1. **While performing a lumbar epidural using a loss of resistance to saline (LORS) technique, you disconnect the syringe from the Tuohy needle to find there is clear fluid very obviously dripping from the needle. What is the best way to confirm whether this fluid is cerebrospinal fluid (CSF)?**
    A. Observe rate and duration of fluid dripping
    B. Assess temperature of fluid with back of gloved hand
    C. Dipstick fluid to determine specific gravity
    D. Send for beta 2 transferrin assay
    E. Dipstick fluid to test for glucose

2. **You review a 28-year-old woman two days post normal vaginal delivery. She received epidural analgesia in labour. She complains of severe postural headache and double vision. On examination she in unable to abduct her left eye. The most likely cause of her symptoms is:**
    A. Cerebral venous thrombosis
    B. Subdural haemorrhage
    C. Migraine
    D. Multiple sclerosis
    E. Dural puncture headache

3. **The most common cause of pregnancy-related death worldwide is:**
    A. Sepsis
    B. Suicide
    C. Haemorrhage
    D. Embolism
    E. Hypertensive disorders

4. **A Jehovah's witness is receiving a transfusion of 200 mL of salvaged blood following an uneventful elective caesarean section. Blood loss during surgery was 400 mL. She suddenly reports feeling unwell. Heart rate is 120 bpm and BP 60/30. The most likely complication of transfusion is:**
   A. ABO incompatibility
   B. Transfusion via leucodepletion filter
   C. Amniotic fluid contamination
   D. Sepsis
   E. Contamination with fetal red cells

5. **Regarding inadvertent dural puncture during labour epidural administration, which of the following has the largest impact on reducing the appearance of headache?**
   A. Higher gauge Tuohy needle
   B. Restriction of pushing
   C. Intrathecal saline administration
   D. Prophylactic epidural blood patch
   E. Supra-normal fluid intake

6. **You are asked to review a 22-year-old woman in early labour. She has a history of hydrocephalus from childhood and a functioning ventriculo-peritoneal shunt** *in situ*. **She has no neurological symptoms. The most correct advice is:**
   A. Epidural analgesia or spinal anaesthesia can be offered as needed
   B. Epidural analgesia can be offered but spinal anaesthesia should be avoided
   C. Epidural analgesia should be avoided but spinal anaesthesia can be offered
   D. Neuraxial techniques are absolutely contraindicated
   E. Discuss caesarean section at the earliest opportunity under general anaesthetic

7. **A 28-year-old primigravida requires lumbar epidural analgesia in labour. During insertion of the epidural a recognized dural puncture occurs with an 18G Tuohy needle. The best way of reducing the incidence of headache now is:**
   A. Injection of intrathecal saline
   B. Insertion of intrathecal catheter and leave in place for 24 hours
   C. Establish epidural analgesia
   D. Intrathecal opioid administration
   E. Prophylactic epidural blood patch

8. **The most common cause of major obstetric haemorrhage is:**
   A. Uterine rupture
   B. Uterine atony
   C. Placental abruption
   D. Placenta praevia
   E. Placenta accreta

9. **A 45-year-old para 4 patient has just delivered a 4.0 kg baby by forceps in theatre. Her epidural has been topped up to provide analgesia. She is having a post-partum haemorrhage. The blood loss is currently 1 L and is ongoing. So far, you have given oxytocin 5 units IV, a further 5 units of oxytocin IV, ergometrine 500 µg IV, one dose of carboprost 250 µg IM. An oxytocin infusion has been commenced. The next best step in the pharmacological management of haemorrhage is:**
   A. Give vitamin K 10 mg IV
   B. Give oral misoprostol 600 µg
   C. Give tranexamic acid 1 g IV
   D. Give recombinant factor VIIa
   E. Give calcium carbonate 10 mmol/L IV

10. **You are asked to review a mother two days post partum complaining of unilateral leg weakness when crossing her legs. She had an epidural sited during first stage of labour before delivery of a 3.3kg baby by mid-cavity forceps. What is the most likely cause of her postpartum neurological deficit?**
    A. Lithotomy position for delivery
    B. Epidural injury
    C. Forceps delivery
    D. Stroke
    E. Descent of fetal head

11. **A 24-year-old primigravida is having a category 4 caesarean section for placenta praevia. She is rhesus negative; 600 mL of blood has been salvaged. What is the most appropriate management regarding infusion of salvaged blood?**
    A. No leukodepletion filter, perform re-crossmatch post transfusion
    B. Use leukodepletion filter, perform Kleihauer test post transfusion
    C. Use leukodepletion filter, perform re-crossmatch post transfusion
    D. Use leukodepletion filter, perform Coomb's test post transfusion
    E. No leukodepletion filter, perform Kleihauer test post transfusion

12. **A primigravida with severe pre-eclampsia on labour ward is 4 cm dilated and requesting an epidural. On admission earlier today her blood pressure was 160/110 mmHg and is currently 140/90 mmHg after oral labetolol. She has significant proteinuria. Her platelet count at her midwife appointment two days ago was 206 $\times$ 10^9/L and on admission earlier today was 141 $\times$ 10^9/L with normal coagulation. What is the best advice for her labour analgesia?**

A. Proceed with epidural

B. Commence Entonox N_2O/O_2. Review need for epidural subsequently

C. Commence 15 mg of IM diamorphine intermittently as required

D. Commence remifentanil PCA

E. Commence morphine patient controlled

13. **You are treating a 26-year-old primigravida who is at 37 weeks' gestation. She has severe pre-eclampsia and is receiving both intravenous magnesium sulphate infusion and labetalol infusion. She now complains of double vision. On examination you note she has a respiratory rate of 12 bpm, BP of 150/90, O$_2$ saturations of 95% on air, and has lost her patellar reflexes. What would be the next step in the pharmacological management of this patient?**

A. Bolus of labetalol

B. Bolus of hydralazine

C. Bolus of lorazepam

D. Bolus of magnesium sulphate

E. Bolus of calcium gluconate 10%

14. **A 25-year old primigravida presents for antenatal anaesthetic assessment at 32 weeks' gestation. She has a history of benign intracranial hypertension which has been asymptomatic. She is otherwise well and has a normal BMI. She is keen for a normal vaginal delivery and wants to discuss her options. You recommend:**

A. Treat as normal

B. Allow labour but avoid all neuraxial blocks for labour and delivery

C. Early labour epidural

D. Elective caesarean section under spinal

E. Elective caesarean section under general anaesthetic

15. **You review a 31-year-old para 1+0 patient in recovery after an isolated BP reading of 75/40 mmHg. She had a category 2 caesarean section under spinal anaesthesia with intrathecal diamorphine, 4 hours earlier, during which she lost 1,500 mL of blood. She complains of mild abdominal discomfort on moving and right shoulder tip pain. Heart rate is 102, respiratory rate 22, and capillary refill time 3 seconds. She is apyrexial and has passed 20 mL of urine postoperatively. What is the most likely cause of her symptoms?**

    A. Sepsis
    B. Pulmonary embolism
    C. Overdose opioid
    D. Hypovolaemia
    E. Blocked catheter

16. **A mother is requesting epidural analgesia during the second stage of labour. She had 10 mg of diamorphine 30 min ago. Her husband is against an epidural as she has written in her birthing plan that she does not want an epidural under any circumstances. What should you do?**

    A. Proceed with the epidural
    B. Not proceed with the epidural and comply with her wishes in her birthing plan
    C. Suggest remifentanil patient-controlled analgesia (PCA) instead
    D. Advise epidural not likely to be effective in time for delivery
    E. Ask the midwife to re-examine the patient

17. **A primiparous 26-year-old lady with BMI 46, presents in spontaneous labour carrying a twin pregnancy. She requests epidural analgesia. On siting this you cause an inadvertent dural tap. The best management of this situation is:**

    A. Abandon procedure, explain to patient, and ask a colleague to resite epidural
    B. Abandon procedure and offer PCA remifentanil
    C. Move needle and site epidural in another space
    D. Give a mini spinal dose of local anaesthetic and discuss options with the patient
    E. Insert the catheter intrathecally and use as a spinal catheter

18. **A 32-year-old primigravida is having an elective caesarean section for breech presentation. On walking in to theatre she develops a regular tachycardia of 210 bpm, the QRS duration is 0.1 seconds. She is fully conscious, aware of unpleasant palpitations, and BP is 90/50. She has a past medical history of supraventricular tachycardia and asthma. Vagal manoeuvres make no difference. The next appropriate management is:**

    A. Amiodarone 300 mg
    B. Adenosine 6 mg
    C. Bisoprolol 2.5 mg
    D. Verapamil 2.5 mg
    E. Digoxin 500 µg

19. **You see an obese primigravida in the obstetric high-risk antenatal clinic. She has a BMI of 44 at present and is 32 weeks' gestation. The best advice to give her for labour and delivery is:**

    A. Recommend elective caesarean section

    B. Recommend PCA remifentanil in labour

    C. Recommend early epidural in labour

    D. Counsel about benefits of losing weight between now and delivery

    E. Counsel about risks of difficult epidural, difficult spinal, failed intubation

20. **You are called to anaesthetize a woman who does not speak English, for a category 2 caesarean section. What is the best way to take a history from and provide information to this patient?**

    A. Professional telephone translation service

    B. The Obstetric Registrar who has some understanding of the patient's language

    C. The patient's husband who has a limited command of English

    D. The patient's 11-year-old daughter, who is bilingual

    E. Written translated materials

1. E

The danger of accidental dural puncture is such that the anaesthetists must be able to diagnose whether it has occurred or not, when suspected by fluid dripping out of the needle.

Further, the diagnosis needs to be made quickly at the bedside to inform ongoing management of the patient and to decide whether a spinal catheter is indicated.

In this scenario the fluid will either be cerebrospinal fluid or saline 0.9% used in the loss of resistance syringe. It is possible to distinguish the two substances by comparison of temperature (subjectively reported using a gloved hand), protein, or glucose estimation on dipstick testing, and by measuring pH value. Cerebrospinal fluid typically will be warm, contain glucose and protein, and have a pH greater around 7.4. 'Normal' saline is relatively acidotic with pH 7.0. Rarely saline may test positive for protein or glucose if it has been contaminated by blood. Assessing temperature of the fluid may be a reliable way to distinguish the two liquids but is subject to variables such as ambient, patient, and operator temperature, etc. An objective test is more reliable than this subjective one. Therefore the best answer in this scenario is dipsticking to test for glucose.

Estimation of free flow rate alone has been shown to be unreliable as a means of distinguishing the two fluids.

Properties of CSF

Specific gravity   1.006–1.008

Opening pressure   90–180 mmH$_2$O

pH 7   28–7.32

Na   135–150 mmol/L

Cl   116–127 mmol/L

Glucose   45–80 mg/dL

Beta 2 transferrin assay is the gold standard test for CSF. This specialized test is carried out in only a few centres in the UK and results may take up to one week to be reported. Indications may include elucidation in a patient complaining of rhinorrhoea for example. Thus it is not useful in the clinical scenario described above given the delays in reporting.

El-Behesy BAZ, James D, Koh KF, et al. Distinguishing CSF from saline used to identify the extradural space. *British Journal of Anaesthesia* 1996; 77: 784–785.

Holloway TE, Telford RJ. Observations on deliberate dural puncture with a Tuohy needle. *Anaesthesia* 1991; 46: 722–724.

2. E

The patient has a sixth nerve (abducens) palsy causing failure of lateral eye movement causing diplopia.

This is the most common cranial nerve palsy after dural puncture associated with intracranial hypotension. The patient also complains of postural headache and had an epidural in labour.

No further information is offered regarding complications during insertion of the epidural. However, this does not exclude a subsequent headache and in fact is a not an infrequent finding. The other causes are rare; however, a pragmatic lower threshold for imaging prior to considering epidural blood patch is recommended due to the presence of new coexisting neurology.

Chambers DJ, Bhatia K. Cranial nerve palsy following central neuraxial block in obstetrics—a review of the literature and analysis of 43 case reports. *International Journal of Obstetric Anesthesia* 2017; 31: 13–26.

3. C

About 830 women die from pregnancy or childbirth-related complications around the world every day. It was estimated that in 2015, approximately 303,000 women died during and following pregnancy and childbirth. Almost all of these deaths occurred in low-resource settings, and most could have been prevented. According to the WHO, haemorrhage accounted for 27.1%, hypertensive disorders 14.0%, and sepsis 10.7% of maternal deaths. The remainder of deaths were due to abortion 7.9%, embolism 3.2%, and all other direct causes of death 9.6%. Regional estimates vary substantially. Haemorrhage is the sixth most common direct cause of maternal death in the UK.

Say L, Chou D, Gemmill A, et al. Global causes of maternal death: a WHO systematic analysis. *Lancet Global Health* 2014; 2 (6): e323–e333.

4. B

Leukodepletion filters are recommended in obstetrics by AAGBI guidance. There have been recent reports of severe hypotension with re-infusion of salvaged blood using leukocyte depletion filters. The mechanism is likely to be bradykinin release and management includes stopping transfusion, removing the filter, and transfusing without the filter. ABO incompatibility is unlikely as the patient is receiving their own blood back and being a Jehovah's witness the extracorporeal circuit would be set up in continuous connection with the patient. Salvaged blood would be unlikely to have become contaminated to cause sepsis during an uncomplicated caesarean and the time frame is one of immediate re-transfusion.

Amniotic fluid is reduced by washing and a two-suction set up. Fetal red cell contamination is reduced by filtration with maternal sensitization for subsequent pregnancies a greater concern.

Cross S, Clark V. Major obstetric haemorrhage. e-LfH https://portal.e-lfh.org.uk/

AAGBI Safety Guideline. Blood transfusion and the anaesthetist. Intra-operative Cell Salvage. September 2009. Available at: https://www.aagbi.org/publications/guidelines/blood-transfusion-and-anaesthetist-intra-operative-cell-salvage

5. A

There is substantial evidence that using a smaller epidural needle (higher gauge, e.g. 18G instead of 16G) reduces the risk and severity of headache. There is a lack of sufficient evidence in support of the other options in the questions.

Paech MJ. Iatrogenic headaches: Giving everyone a sore head (editorial). *International Journal Obstetric Anesthesia* 2012; 21: 1–3.

6. A

If the shunt is functioning normally as suggested by an absence of symptoms of hydrocephalus, then both neuraxial techniques have been used and can be offered. Vaginal delivery is the preferred route in women with a functioning shunt. However, neuraxial techniques in women with shunt failure are generally considered to be contraindicated and could increase the risk of brain herniation. Caesarean section is indicated with shunt failure and raised ICP.

Caesarean delivery may also potentially damage the peritoneal part of the shunt.

Rajagopalan S, Gopinath S, Trinh VT, Chandrasekhar S. Anesthetic considerations for labor and delivery in women with cerebrospinal fluid shunts. *International Journal of Obstetric Anesthesia* 2017; 30: 23–29.

7. B

Various strategies to prevent the onset of headache have been used such as prophylactic epidural blood patch (EBP) or intrathecal saline injection. The most widely practiced is that of inserting an intrathecal catheter at the time of dural puncture. Study results are conflicting but suggest that most benefit occurs when the catheter is left in place for 24 hours. A recent meta-analysis demonstrated a significant reduction in the incidence of post dural puncture headache (PDPH) from 66% to 51% and requirement for EBP from 59% to 33% after intrathecal catheter placement.

However, the monitoring and procedures in place to ensure safety of this practice in an individual unit is of paramount importance and should also be considered.

Van de Velde M, Schepers R, Berends N, et al. Ten years of experience with accidental dural puncture and post-dural puncture headache in tertiary obstetric anaesthesia department. *International Journal of Obstetric Anesthesia* 2008; 17: 329–335.

8. B

Although blood loss may be concealed or difficult to measure, fetal distress, loss of uterine tone, and rising abdominal girth may indicate ongoing blood loss. The majority of bleeds are post-partum and caused by uterine atony. Many of the other causes of haemorrhage are also a risk factor for uterine atony.

S. Cross, V. Clark. Major Obstetric Haemorrhage e-LfH.

9. C

The post-partum haemorrhage is most likely due to uterine atony as she is multiparous and has delivered a large baby. In addition, there may be trauma to the birth canal following delivery.

Tranexamic acid has been shown to be beneficial in the management of post-partum haemorrhage. Although it is not yet clear if this finding will be transferable to a UK cohort it remains the best answer as all others can be excluded as being less useful.

To be of benefit, it must be given as soon as possible after the haemorrhage is diagnosed: 1 g is given initially with a further 1 g given 30 min later.

Oral or PR misoprostol can be given in the absence of intravenous access or if there are no supplies of the IV drug preparations.

Recombinant factor VIIa is used in the prevention and treatment of bleeding due to haemophilia.

Vitamin K is indicated to reverse warfarin therapy Calcium replacement may be required during subsequent blood transfusion.

Shakur H, Roberts I, Fawole B et al. Effect of early tranexamic acid administration on mortality, hysterectomy, and other morbidities in women with post-partum haemorrhage (WOMAN): an international, randomised, double-blind, placebo-controlled trial. Lancet 2017; 389 (10084): 2105–2116.

WHO guidelines for managing post-partum haemorrhage. Available at: http://apps.who.int/iris/bitstream/10665/75411/1/9789241548502_eng.pdf

10. C

She has an obturator nerve palsy. Obstetric causes most likely. The classic feature is weakness of leg adduction (difficulty crossing legs) with a patch of numbness on the inner aspect of thigh if examined. Women presenting with neurological dysfunction in the post-partum period may have symptoms secondary to either complications of regional anaesthesia or obstetric nerve injury. The overall incidence of major complications resulting in permanent harm following central neuraxial blockade (spinal and/or epidural block) in the obstetric population is 1 in 80,000 to 1 in 320,000. Clinically important transient neurological dysfunction from an obstetric cause is estimated to be 1 in 500, i.e. much more common.

Lithotomy position can lead to foot drop due to compression of common peroneal nerve by the stirrups. Stroke is rare and likely to produce a central nerve lesion deficit, e.g. hemiparesis.

A common cause of problems is the fetal head compressing the lumbosacral trunk where it crosses the posterior pelvic brim before descending in front of the sacral ala. Usually, however, this causes femoral nerve symptoms with limited quadriceps strength and also reduced hip flexion. Foot drop can be a notable consequence of these mechanics too. The foot drop is almost always unilateral and on the opposite side to the fetal occiput resulting in weak dorsiflexion and eversion with decreased sensation on the lateral lower leg and dorsal foot.

Boyce H, Plaat F. Post-natal neurological problems. *Continuing Education in Anaesthesia Critical Care & Pain* 2013; 13 (20) 63–66.

National Audit Project (NAP) 3. The Royal College of Anaesthetists January 2009: Major complications of central neuraxial block in the United Kingdom.

https://www.rcoa.ac.uk/system/files/CSQ-NAP3-results-presentation.pdf

11. B

Concerns about amniotic fluid embolism, rhesus sensitization, and fetal debris contamination previously limited the use of cell salvage in obstetric practice. However, to date, there have been no proven cases of amniotic fluid embolism caused by reinfusion of salvaged blood in the literature. The utilization of leucodepletion filters during transfusion of salvaged blood can reduce the fetal squamous cell contamination to a level comparable with maternal blood contamination. However, it is not recommended that salvaged blood be pressurized through these filters as it may cause hypotension from the release of vasoactive substances such as bradykinin.

The cell saver cannot distinguish fetal from maternal red cells. If the mother is rhesus negative (and the fetus RhD positive) the extent of maternal exposure should be determined by Kleihauer testing as soon as possible and a suitable dose of anti-D immunoglobulin given (usually 125 IU/mL of fetal blood).

AAGBI Safety Guideline. Blood transfusion and the anaesthetist. Intra-operative Cell Salvage. September 2009. Available at: https://www.aagbi.org/publications/guidelines/blood-transfusion-and-anaesthetist-intra-operative-cell-salvage

Association of Anaesthetists of Great Britain and Ireland. AAGBI guidelines: the use of blood components and their alternatives 2016. *Anaesthesia* 2016; 71: 829–842.

Kuppurao L, Wee M. Perioperative cell salvage. *Continuing Education in Anaesthesia Critical Care & Pain* 2010; 10 (4): 104–108.

12. A

An epidural technique will help control blood pressure and improve placental blood flow. It will also allow conversion to epidural anaesthesia if assisted or operative delivery required. This is superior to IM opioid and preferable to remifentanil in this case. PCA morphine is not suitable for labour pain due to its kinetics and Entonox will provide only low grade analgesia leaving blood pressure susceptible to surges with contraction pain. Her platelet count has had a modest fall over a period of days which is not obviously precipitous. It is still at a level where epidural can be reasonably considered.

Hart E, Coley S. The diagnosis and management of pre-eclampsia. *BJA CEPD Reviews* 2003; 3 (2): 38–42.

NICE Guideline. Clinical Guideline CG 107 published August 2010 Updated January 2011 Hypertension in pregnancy: Diagnosis and management. Available at: https://www.nice.org.uk/guidance/cg107/chapter/1-guidance

13. E

This patient is exhibiting signs of hypermagnesaemia and the management would be to stop magnesium infusion and give calcium.

The other options are treatments for pre-eclampsia/eclampsia.

Hart E, Coley S. The diagnosis and management of pre-eclampsia. *BJA CEPD Reviews* 2003; 3 (2): 38–42.

Paterson-Brown S, Howell C. *Managing Obstetric Emergencies and Trauma.* Cambridge: Cambridge University Press 2016.

14. C

Benign intracranial hypertension is a diagnosis of exclusion described as raised intracranial pressure (ICP) in the absence of an intracranial lesion, hydrocephalus or infection, and normal cerebrospinal fluid (CSF) composition. Patients usually present with headache characteristic of raised ICP, visual disturbance, and nausea. The condition is more common in obese women while symptoms often worsen during pregnancy and improve after delivery. Symptomatic patients are at risk of further compromise if allowed to labour due to an increase in CSF and epidural pressures during uterine contractions and the second stage of labour. Asymptomatic patients should be offered effective regional analgesia and an elective instrumental will reduce surges in ICP.

Griffiths S, Durbridge JA. Anaesthetic implications of neurological disease in pregnancy. *Continuing Education in Anaesthesia Critical Care & Pain* 2011; 11 (5): 157–161.

15. D

This is a common clinical picture in recovery in obstetrics and ongoing bleeding must be suspected. Blood pressure is well maintained in otherwise fit adults until compensation is no longer possible. At this stage 30–40% of circulating blood volume has been lost. Any episode of hypotension should be taken seriously.

The patient's signs are consistent with hypovolaemia. (tachycardia, hypotension, increased respiratory rate, and prolonged capillary refill time). A full blood count will help differentiate between a lack of fluid intake and occult intra-abdominal bleeding. Sepsis should be considered post caesarean section but would usually be accompanied by pyrexia or hypothermia. Full blood count will provide estimation of neutrophil count. Her low urine output is worrying and serum urea and electrolytes should be checked and the catheter flushed to exclude obstruction. However, catheter obstruction and bladder distension would cause a raised blood pressure and constant discomfort.

Her respiratory rate is raised making opioid overdose unlikely.

Act for Libraries. Medical Science. Indications of post-operative bleeding. Available at: http://www. actforlibraries.org/indications-of-post-op-bleeding-or-signs-of-post-op-bleeding/

Carle C, Alexander P, Columb M, et al. Design and internal validation of an obstetric early warning score: Secondary analysis of the Intensive Care National Audit and Research Centre Case Mix Programme database. *Anaesthesia* 2013; 68 354–367.

Martin RL. Midwives' experiences of using a modified early obstetric warning score (MEOWS): A grounded theory study. *Evidence Based Midwifery* 2015; 13 (2): 59–65.

Singh S, McGlennan A, England A, et al. A validation study of the CEMACH recommended modified early obstetric warning system (MEOWS). *Anaesthesia* 2012; 67: 12–18.

16. E

It does not matter what is written in the birthing plan, the patient can change her mind. No partner, or other adult without power of attorney, can give or withhold consent on behalf of another adult.

Remifentanil PCA is relatively contraindicated so soon after pethidine. Second stage of labour begins when the cervix is fully dilated. As it can last for a variable length of time an epidural may or may not prove helpful to an individual patient and may even assist in relaxing the pelvic floor or assisted delivery. It's appropriate to request more information in the form of an examination to help direct judgements regarding appropriateness of epidural intervention.

A or E are acceptable but it would be better to check she is not actually about to imminently deliver before siting epidural so there is some benefit present to balance the accepted risks of the procedure.

Jackson GN, Sensky T, Reide P, Yentis SM. The capacity to consent to epidural analgesia in labour. *International Journal of Obstetric Anesthesia* 2011; 20 (3): 269–270.

Middle JV, Wee MYK. Informed consent for epidural analgesia in labour: a survey of UK practice. *Anaesthesia* 2009; 64: 161–164.

17. E

This parturient requires effective analgesia that can be adapted for assisted delivery and caesarean section if necessary.

No particular acute management of a dural tap reduces the incidence of headache, and having accepted the risks of the procedure it is preferable to deliver the proposed benefit, of good pain relief, to the woman also. This can be provided by a spinal catheter, clearly labelled as such, and only to be topped up by the duty anaesthetist.

Baraz R, Collis RE. The management of accidental dural puncture during labour epidural analgesia: a survey of UK practice. *Anaesthesia* 2005; 60: 673–679.

Deng J, Wang L, Zhang L, et al. Insertion of an intrathecal catheter in parturients reduces the risk of post-dural puncture headache: A retrospective study and meta-analysis. PLoS One 2017; 12 (7): e0180504.

18. D

There are no significant adverse features warranting immediate synchronized DC cardioversion. If there were adverse features present it may still be appropriate to attempt vagal manoeuvres or immediate drug treatment to terminate an SVT. Amiodarone is a recognized treatment but not first line, and although described in pregnancy there are concerns regarding side effect profile and crossing the placenta. Adenosine is relatively contraindicated by asthma. Bisoprolol may be used prophylactically to reduce the frequency/severity of palpitations but is again relatively contraindicated by asthma.

Verapamil 2.5–5 mg can be used intravenously acutely to terminate SVT when adenosine is contraindicated. Digoxin has a relatively slower onset and is more appropriate in an irregular narrow complex tachycardia, e.g. atrial fibrillation.

Resuscitation Council (UK). Peri-arrest arrhythmias. Available at: https://www.resus.org.uk/resuscitation-guidelines/peri-arrest-arrhythmias/

19. C

C is the most sensible and practical advice to give. An epidural will be easier to site than waiting until labour is advanced. It can be assessed for top-up potential should operative delivery be required and confirmation that it is working well reduces the likelihood of general anaesthesia being required.

Weight loss is unlikely to be achieved nor make a significant difference to anaesthetic interventions and dieting during the third trimester should not be recommended by the anaesthetist.

Opting for elective caesarean section is a decision for obstetricians. Nonetheless, it is not an easy option. The risks for the mother are slightly higher and it is more likely she will have repeat caesarean sections with subsequent pregnancies complicated by post-partum haemorrhage.

Arabin B, Stupin JH. Overweight and obesity before, during and after Pregnancy: Part 2: Evidence-based risk factors and interventions. *Geburtshilfe und Frauenheilkunde*. 2014; 74 (7): 646–655.

Arrowsmith S, Wray S, Quenby S. Maternal obesity and labour complications following induction of labour in prolonged pregnancy. *BJOG* 2011; 118 (5): 578–588.

Gupta A, Faber P. Obesity in pregnancy. *Continuing Education in Anaesthesia Critical Care & Pain* 2011; 11 (4): 143–146.

Panni MK, Columb MO. Obese parturients have lower epidural local anaesthetic requirements for analgesia in labour. *British Journal of Anaesthesia* 2006; 96 (1): 106–110.

20. A

While delivery is expedited, there is time to take an adequate history for a category 2 caesarean section as there is deemed no immediate threat to life of mother or baby. Medical information should be sought and given to a patient by an independent party. If time allows a professional translator should be requested to attend to allow a two-way conversation but if the situation is urgent a telephone translation service is the next best option (answer A). Accurate translation is important as the patient must be fully informed in order to give or withhold consent. This onerous role should not be entrusted to a minor or anyone with less than fluent grasp of the patient's first language including medical terminology.

Written material can be given in the patient's native language. However, these do not help us establish the patient's past medical history or allow question and answer clarification with the clinician.

Royal College of Obstetricians and Gynaecologists. *Safer Childbirth. Minimum Standards for the Organisation and Delivery of Care in Labour.* London: RCOG. Available at: www.rcog.org.uk

1. **You review a hypotensive patient in intensive care. The arterial line trace appears over-damped. In order to improve the waveform the next action is:**
   A. Examine tubing for air bubbles
   B. Flush the tubing and catheter
   C. Lengthen the tubing
   D. Use wider diameter tubing
   E. Reinsert arterial line

2. **You perform an internal jugular central line on an adult under ultrasound guidance. The ultrasound machine has a number of probes attached. Which is the best ultrasound probe to use?**
   A. Hockey stick footprint
   B. Linear array
   C. Curvilinear array
   D. Micro curvilinear array
   E. Phased array

3. **Regarding severe community-acquired pneumonia. The best risk stratification tool for identifying patients who may require invasive respiratory support in critical care is:**
   A. SMART-COP
   B. CURB-65
   C. Pneumonia Severity Index (PSI)
   D. APACHE II
   E. Severe Community Acquired Pneumonia Score

4. **A 30-year-old woman presents to the ED having taken an overdose of 16 paracetamol tablets with half a bottle of vodka about three hours ago. She has a history of epilepsy for which she has been on long-term phenytoin. She is crying and saying she doesn't want to die. The most effective initial management would be?**

    A. Once paracetamol level available and confirmed as toxic start treatment with N-acetyl cysteine
    B. Start N-acetyl cysteine treatment immediately
    C. Give activated charcoal orally and then once paracetamol level back treat with N-acetyl cysteine if required
    D. Perform gastric lavage and then if paracetamol level toxic treat with N-acetyl cysteine
    E. Start N-acetyl cysteine treatment immediately and perform haemodialysis as soon as possible

5. **A 59-year-old man is on airway pressure release ventilation (APRV) mode of ventilation for respiratory failure. The current ventilatory settings are FiO_2 = 0.4, P high = 30 cmH_2O, P low = 0 cm H_2O, T high = 4.8 s, and T low = 0.8 s. He is not oversedated and is making good spontaneous respiratory effort. His pCO_2 is 11.1 and his pO_2 is 12.9 on his last arterial blood gas. How would you best adjust the ventilator settings to now?**

    A. Set termination of expiration flow to 90% maximum
    B. Increase the FiO_2 to 0.6
    C. Increase the P low by 5 cmH_2O
    D. Decrease the P high by 2 cmH_2O
    E. Increase the P high by 2 cmH_2O

6. **A 71-year-old lady is in ICU for management of severe respiratory failure secondary to community acquired pneumonia. She has been ventilated for eight days and her ventilatory settings are an FiO_2 of 0.9 and a PEEP of 10 cmH_2O. This has not improved despite a trial of prone positioning. Which of the following would be a contraindication to extracorporeal membrane oxygenation (ECMO) in this patient?**

    A. Presence of a bronchopleural fistula
    B. FiO_2 >0.8 for >7 days
    C. Age >65
    D. Four quadrant infiltrates on her chest X-ray
    E. Murray score >3

7. **A 52-year-old man in ICU required intubation and ventilation three days ago following aspiration of gastric contents. He has bilateral infiltrates on his chest X-ray and a PaO$_2$/FiO$_2$ ratio of <200 mmHg. You decide to try prone ventilation. Which statement best describes ventilation in the prone position?**

   A. The patient must have an infusion of muscle relaxant
   B. Carbon dioxide clearance is usually decreased
   C. Oxygenation is improved by reducing anatomical dead space
   D. It improves patient survival
   E. It is contraindicated in patients requiring renal replacement therapy

8. **An unknown adult male is presented to the emergency department by ambulance with GCS 10. He has multi-organ failure and is in need of organ support. There is no history from the patient. His initial results reveal:**

   Na$^+$ 150 mmol/L
   K$^+$ 6.0 mmol/L
   Cl$^-$ 106 mmol/L
   HCO$_3^-$ 13 mmol/L
   Urea 38 mmol/L
   Creat 467 μmol/L
   H$^+$ 78 nmol/L
   pO$_2$ 12.1 kPa
   pCO$_2$ 2.4 kPa
   HCO$_3$ 13 mmol/L. Which potential diagnosis can be excluded?

   A. Salicylate poisoning
   B. Severe diarrhoea
   C. Rhabdomyolysis
   D. Ethylene glycol poisoning
   E. Diabetic ketoacidosis

9. **The ICU you are working in uses citrate as the method of providing anticoagulation for renal replacement therapy (RRT) instead of intravenous heparin infusion. What is the main advantage of using citrate for anticoagulation in this clinical situation?**

   A. Avoids need for protocolized infusion
   B. Less metabolic disturbance
   C. Avoids systemic anticoagulation
   D. Causes less disturbance of calcium levels
   E. Reduced risk of embolic complications

10. **A 68-year-old male is admitted to intensive care with sepsis causing multi-organ failure. He requires central venous access for a low-dose noradrenaline (norepinephrine) infusion which is currently running through a peripheral cannula. His blood results reveal platelets 62 and INR 1.6. The most appropriate action is:**

    A. Proceed to femoral line by most experienced operator
    B. Platelet transfusion before internal jugular line
    C. Platelet transfusion and fresh frozen plasma before internal jugular
    D. Platelet transfusion and fresh frozen plasma before subclavian line
    E. Proceed to internal jugular line by most experienced operator

11. **You have intubated a 43-year-old male who presented to the Emergency Department having been rescued from a fire in his living room. He had lost consciousness at the scene and smelt strongly of alcohol. He had minor burns but had soot in his nose and mouth and a carboxyhaemoglobin level of 22%. What is the most important intervention to improve outcome?**

    A. Prone ventilation
    B. Early administration of steroids
    C. Early bronchoscopy and washout
    D. Prophylactic antibiotics
    E. Regular nebulized heparin and acetyl cysteine

12. **A 36-year-old brainstem dead patient is in ITU awaiting organ harvest. He suffered a traumatic brain injury. He is 70 kg. The urine output is 400 mL/hour for the last 3 hours. The serum sodium is 155 mmol/L, serum osmolality is 321 mosmol/kg, and urine osmolality is 120 mosmol/kg. The most likely diagnosis is:**

    A. SIADH (syndrome of inappropriate antidiuretic hormone secretion)
    B. Cerebral salt wasting
    C. Dehydration/hypovolaemia
    D. Furosemide administration
    E. Diabetes insipidus

13. **A 39-year-old woman presents with a two-day history of gradual onset weakness. She had an upper respiratory tract infection two weeks ago but is otherwise well. Clinical examination elicits symmetrical reduction in tone and power in all four limbs which is worse in the upper limbs than the lower limbs. What is the most likely diagnosis?**

    A. Myasthenia Gravis
    B. Eaton–Lambert syndrome
    C. Multiple sclerosis
    D. Guillain–Barré syndrome
    E. Critical care neuropathy

14. **A previously fit and well 21-year-old female presents to the Emergency Department having taken ecstasy tablets. Her temperature is 40.1°C and she has been fitting. She has a GCS of 5 prior to intubation and you have commenced cooling measures. Her sodium level is 114 mmol/L. The best way to treat this hyponatraemia is:**
    A. Give hypertonic saline 3%
    B. Give furosemide
    C. Give demeclocycline
    D. Start haemofiltration
    E. Give normal saline

15. **A 69-year-old female presents to the Emergency Department with fever, dyspnoea, a productive cough, and right sided pleuritic chest pain. A chest X-ray confirms a right middle lobe pneumonia. The most likely infective pathogen in this case is:**
    A. *Haemophilus influenza*
    B. *Legionella*
    C. *Streptococcus pneumoniae*
    D. *Klebsiella pneumoniae*
    E. Influenza A virus

16. **A 60-year-old male with an exacerbation of chronic obstructive pulmonary disease has required ventilation in the Intensive Care Unit for 18 days. He is proving difficult to wean from the ventilator. He is sedated with a propofol infusion, but with any reduction in the infusion rate he becomes intolerant of the endotracheal tube and coughs persistently. The best strategy to increase the chances of weaning successfully is:**
    A. Stop propofol, extubate, and assess. Reintubate if necessary
    B. Start a morphine infusion before reducing propofol
    C. Start a remifentanil infusion before reducing propofol
    D. Start a dexmedetomidine infusion
    E. Transfer to theatre for a surgical tracheostomy

17. **You admit a patient with pneumonia and respiratory failure to ICU and start enteral feeding as part of your general management. Which of the following factors confer the highest risk of refeeding syndrome?**
    A. Body mass index (BMI) of 18 kg/m^2
    B. Chronic alcohol abuse
    C. A potassium level of 3.3 mmol/L prior to feeding
    D. Unintentional weight loss of 10% in the last six months
    E. Minimal nutritional intake for 15 days

18. **A 63-year-old female is declared brainstem dead following a massive intracranial bleed. She is now being optimized for organ harvest in your ICU. Her blood pressure is 81/45 mmHg despite fluid resuscitation. What would be the next step in cardiovascular management?**

    A. Start a vasopressin infusion
    B. Give a bolus of methylprednisolone
    C. Start an infusion of thyroid hormone T3
    D. Start a noradrenaline (norepinephrine) infusion
    E. Start an adrenaline (epinephrine) infusion

19. **An ICU patient has a pleural effusion noted on chest X-ray. You perform a diagnostic tap. The biochemistry of the pleural fluid reveals a lactate dehydrogenase of 510 U/L (serum normal range 250–540), pH 7.1, and a glucose of 1.2 mmol/L. The most likely cause of the effusion is:**

    A. Pancreatitis
    B. Congestive heart failure
    C. Nephrotic syndrome
    D. Empyema
    E. Cirrhosis

20. **A 27-year-old woman presents with breathlessness and generalized weakness of rapid onset over 48 hours. Her only history is of chronic intravenous drug misuse. On examination she has fixed dilated pupils, diplopia, ptosis, symmetrical flaccid paralysis of arms/neck, and normal sensation. She is afebrile. The most likely diagnosis is:**

    A. Botulism
    B. Guillain–Barré syndrome
    C. Myasthenia Gravis
    D. Viral encephalitis
    E. Eaton–Lambert syndrome

1. A

Some damping is a feature of every arterial line system and is useful in counteracting the amount of resonance, i.e. optimal damping. It acts to slow down the rate of change of signal between the patient and pressure transducer. An over-damped trace can be caused by occlusion such as kinks or clots, a bubble interrupting the saline column, or using a soft cannula and tubing. The anaesthetist should first check for air and clots. before flushing any line. Lengthening or widening the tubing will worsen the damping. Ultimately it may be appropriate to reinsert the arterial line if the trace cannot be improved.

Ward M, Langton JA. Blood pressure measurement. *Continuing Education in Anaesthesia Critical Care & Pain* 2007; 7 (4): 122–126.

2. B

In general, the higher the frequency of probe, the better the resolution of image but always at the expense of depth of penetration into the body. The target in question is relatively superficial to the skin's surface which indicates that a high-frequency probe should be used in order to give a high-resolution image with shallow penetration. The linear probe can be placed flat on the neck and has a high frequency (6–13 MHz). A phased array is more useful for moving structures such as in echocardiography. A curvilinear probe is of lower frequency (2–5 MHz) allowing deeper examinations such as abdominal ultrasound. A hockey stick has a small footprint and is useful in paediatrics.

Carty S, Nicholls B, Ultrasound-guided regional anaesthesia, *Continuing Education in Anaesthesia Critical Care & Pain* 2007; 7 (1): 20–24.

3. A

Pneumonia Severity Score Index and BTS CURB-65 have been more extensively validated to recognize low-risk patients and are not good at predicting need for critical care support.

SMART-COP and Pneumonia Severity Index perform well in identifying patients who require ICU admission. SMART-COP was created to identify patients who may require respiratory or vasopressor support, a score of 3 or more identifies 92% of those who will require intensive respiratory support.

Charles PG, Wolfe R, Whitby M, et al. SMART-COP: A tool for predicting the need for intensive respiratory support or vasopressor support in community-acquired pneumonia. *Clinical Infectious Diseases* 2008; 47: 375–384.

4. A

The patient has ingested 8,000 mg of paracetamol. This is 100 mg/kg. The paracetamol guidance changed in 2012, made by the Commission for Human Medicines.

A significant ingestion is that above 75 mg/kg, which therefore necessities medical assessment.

Activated charcoal is only useful within 1 hour of ingestion and the calculated dose should be above 150 mg/kg. Lavage is not indicated.

Assessment of liver risk, i.e. alcohol or other medication is no longer required having been removed from most recent guidance to simplify them. Risk factors for paracetamol toxicity (e.g. starvation, hepatic enzyme induction) have previously been used for risk stratification. However, not all are well characterized and they have not always been applied consistently. For this reason, the Commission for Human Medicines has advised that the presence of risk factors should no longer be considered in assessing risk of toxicity after a single acute overdose.

This patient has an accurate history of single overdose within 3 hours. Guidance suggests to wait for the 4-hour paracetamol level before starting N-acetyl cysteine.

If the patient is at risk, i.e. above single treatment line on graph give intravenous acetyl cysteine. There is normally no indication to start acetyl cysteine without a paracetamol blood concentration provided the result can be obtained and acted upon within 8 hours of ingestion.

If there is going to be undue delay in obtaining the paracetamol concentration, treatment should be started if more than 150 mg/kg paracetamol has been ingested.

Treating paracetamol overdose with intravenous acetylcysteine: new guidance. Available at: https://www.gov.uk/drug-safety-update/treating-paracetamol-overdose-with-intravenous-acetylcysteine-new-guidance

5. E

Airway pressure release ventilation is commonly used in the ICU setting to treat ARDS and other conditions associated with severe hypoxia and low compliance. Its advantages include lower airway pressures, lower minute ventilation, and ability to breathe spontaneously throughout ventilatory cycle.

When starting APRV the termination of expiration flow should be set to 75% and this can be decreased towards 50% if hypercarbia is a problem. Increasing FiO_2 will have no effect on CO_2. P low should always be kept at zero to allow minimal resistance to exhalation.

Increasing P high to 40 cmH$_2$O and then increasing T high in 0.5 increments up to 8 seconds would provide best chances of controlling CO_2.

If increasing P high and T high has not worked then increasing the T low to allow more time for alveolar emptying may help.

Milo Frawley P, Habashi NM. Airway pressure release ventilation –theory and practice. *AACN Clinical Issues* 2001; 12; 234–246.

6. B

ECMO is contraindicated when there has been high-pressure ventilation with peak inspiratory pressure >30 cmH$_2$O for >7 days or high FiO_2 for >7 days.

ECMO is also contraindicated if there is an acute or recent intracranial bleed because it requires anticoagulation.

The Murray score is used when considering referral and a score >3 would be a reason for referral. Scores are given for number of chest X-ray quadrants infiltrated, PaO_2/FiO_2 (P/F) ratio, level of PEEP and compliance.

ECMO is indicated for potentially reversible causes of severe respiratory failure including those with a bronchopleural fistula and when there has been failure of prone ventilation.

Age is not a contraindication to ECMO.

Zwischenberger, JB, Lynch JE. Will CESAR answer the adult ECMO debate? *Lancet* Volume 2009; 374 (9698): 1307–1308.

7. D

The patient does not need to be paralysed to tolerate the prone position.

Carbon dioxide clearance is usually increased.

Oxygenation is improved by enhancing alveolar recruitment and reducing ventilation/perfusion mismatch while also reducing overdistension of lung areas. Prone ventilation does not alter anatomical dead space.

The PROSEVA trial demonstrated that in severe ARDS, early and prolonged prone positioning was associated with significant decrease in 28- and 90-day mortality.

It is not contraindicated in patients with RRT although care must be taken with line position.

Guérin C, Reignier J, Richard JC, et al.; for the PROSEVA Study Group. Prone positioning in severe acute respiratory distress syndrome. *New England Journal of Medicine* 2013; 368: 2159–2168.

8. B

This patient has a metabolic acidosis with a raised anion gap of 37 mEq/L (normal range 5–12; anion gap = $[Na^+] + [K^+] - ([Cl^-] - [HCO_3^-])$). Severe diarrhoea results in a loss of bicarbonate and a normal anion gap. All the others provide an additional source of acid which raises the anion Gap.

Grice A. Acid base disorders in critical care–Part 1. Anaesthetic tutorial of the week 66. Available at: http://www.totow.anaesthesiologists.org

9. C

Systemic heparin anticoagulation is the most commonly used method; however, patients are at risk of haemorrhage. Heparin resistance and heparin-induced thrombocytopenia mean alternative forms of anticoagulation must be available.

Citrate's main advantage is that it provides regional anticoagulation within the RRT circuit and avoids the risks mentioned above.

Citrate chelates calcium and therefore platelet aggregation and coagulation. Most of the citrate–calcium complex is removed in the effluent so systemic calcium infusion is often necessary to avoid hypocalcaemia. It can also cause acidosis, alkalosis, and hypomagnesaemia. There must be protocols to monitor and manage these metabolic disturbances.

While using citrate patients will still need prophylaxis against deep venous thrombosis.

Hall NA, Fox AJ. Renal replacement therapies in critical care. *Continuing Education in Anaesthesia Critical Care & Pain* 2006; 6 (5): 197–202.

10. A

In the presence of a coagulopathy, the more experienced operator available should insert the central venous catheter (CVC), ideally at an insertion site that allows easy compression of vessels. Femoral access may have a lower risk in this situation. Routine reversal of coagulopathy is only necessary if platelet count <50 × 109 L⁻¹, activated partial thromboplastin time >1.3 times normal, and/or international normalized ratio >1.8, as the risk of haemorrhage is otherwise not increased. Waiting for arrival of blood products and subsequent transfusion will create delay in the ongoing management of this patient. Peripheral noradrenaline (norepinephrine) in this patient should be regarded as short term before definitive access. In selected patients, different thresholds for correction may be acceptable. Bleeding risks of insertion and removal vary with the site, size of device, and operator experience. The risks of correction (e.g. infection, lung injury, thrombosis) may exceed that of local bleeding, and it may be preferable to give blood products if problems occur, rather than prophylactically.

Association of Anaesthetists of Great Britain and Ireland. Safe vascular access 2016. *Anaesthesia* 2016; 71: 573–585.

11. C

Early bronchoscopy diagnoses and grades the severity of inhalational injury and evidence suggests improved outcomes with bronchoscopy and early clearance of particulate matter and washout. Lung protective strategies as per ARDS guidelines would be common sense but there is little evidence to support this or prone ventilation. An inhalational protocol with nebulized heparin and acetyl cysteine may be of benefit but no large trials support its widespread adoption. There is no place for prophylactic antibiotics. Steroids are not recommended in treatment but may have a role in preventing post-extubation stridor caused by laryngeal oedema.

Gill P, Martin RV. Smoke inhalation injury. *Continuing Education in Anaesthesia Critical Care & Pain* 2015; 15 (3): 143–148.

12. E

Diabetes insipidus. The diuresis is >4 mL/kg. This patient has a resultant high serum sodium (>145 mmol/L), increased serum osmolality (>300), and a reduced urine osmolality (<200). It is due to excess water loss from the body. Fluid replacement with enteral or IV solutions containing minimal sodium needs to treat both fluid deficit and ongoing losses. Early use of vasopressin may prevent the need for additional treatment, but if diabetes insipidus persists, desmopressin is indicated.

SIADH and cerebral salt wasting are associated with hyponatraemia. The primary distinction between cerebral salt wasting and SIADH is volume status. SIADH = fluid retention, low urine output, serum <135, serum osmolality <275, urine osmolality > serum osmolality, high urinary sodium (>25 mEq/L). In cerebral salt wasting the primary pathogenic mechanism is renal loss of sodium, which leads to hyponatraemia and a decrease in extracellular volume. Indications of volume depletion (hypotension, weight loss, and decreased skin turgor) occur with cerebral salt wasting, whereas indications of volume expansion occur with SIADH (decreased urine output and generalized weight gain due to fluid retention). Signs and symptoms are remarkably similar; however, patients with cerebral salt wasting experiences a true loss of sodium and intravascular fluid. Both sodium and fluid must be replaced to correct the imbalance. In patients with SIADH, sodium is replaced, but fluid is restricted.

Gordon JK, McKinlay J. Physiological changes after brain stem death and management of the heart-beating donor. *Continuing Education in Anaesthesia Critical Care & Pain* 2012 12 (5): 225–229.

13. D

The time scale, history of preceding minor viral illness, and clinical findings support a diagnosis of Guillain–Barré syndrome.

Daniel S, Green R. Guillain-Barré syndrome. Anaesthetic Tutorial of the Week 238. Available at: https://www.aagbi.org/sites/default/files/238%20Guillain%20Barre%20Syndrome.pdf

14. A

Severe hyponatraemia can occur due to over-ingestion of water and can lead to cerebral oedema. Given that this is due to a rapid change in sodium concentration it can be reversed quickly.

When hyponatraemia has occurred slowly it must be corrected in a controlled manner to prevent central pontine demyelination.

Roberts TN, Thompson JP. Illegal substances in anaesthetic and intensive care practices. *Continuing Education in Anaesthesia Critical Care & Pain* 2013; 13 (2): 42–46.

15. C

All of these pathogens can cause community-acquired pneumonia but *Streptococcus pneumoniae* is the most common aetiological agent in the UK.

Sadashivaiah JB, Carr B. Severe community-acquired pneumonia. *Continuing Education in Anaesthesia Critical Care & Pain* 2009; 9 (3): 87–91.

16. D

Dexmedetomidine is indicated for light sedation on intensive care as a bridge to extubation. It does not cause respiratory depression nor airway compromise and patients sedated with it are more cooperative and better able to obey commands. It also depresses the gag reflex and improves tracheal tube tolerance compared to other sedative agents and can facilitate a smooth non-combative extubation.

A failed extubation will cause significant setback for the patient. Morphine will reduce respiratory drive and CO_2 responsiveness. Remifentanil, an ultra-short-acting opioid, can be helpful to facilitate extubation but must be titrated exactly and stopped immediately post extubation to avoid airway obstruction, apnoea, and oversedation.

A surgical tracheostomy is a more invasive procedure, better performed in the early days of admission to intensive care.

Scott-Warren VL, Sebastian J. Dexmedetomidine: its use in intensive care medicine and anaesthesia. *BJA Education* 201616 (7): 242–246.

17. E

Little or no nutritional intake for greater than 15 days confers severe high risk of developing refeeding syndrome. As does a BMI <14 kg/m^2.

A BMI <16 kg/m^2, unintentional weight loss of >15% in the previous three to six months, and low levels of potassium, magnesium, or phosphate prior to feeding confer high risk. A history of alcohol abuse or drug therapy with insulin or chemotherapy agents confer moderate risk.

Tomlin G. Refeeding syndrome. Anaesthesia UK. Available at: http://www.frca.co.uk/article.aspx?articleid=100777

18. A

Early use of a vasopressor helps haemodynamic stability and reduces risk of excess fluid administration. Vasopressin is considered the first-line agent where hypotension is resistant to fluid therapy. It is less likely to cause myocardial damage metabolic acidosis or pulmonary hypertension than other inotropes. Thyroid hormone may improve cardiac function but its benefit is questionable.

Gordon, J McKinlay J. Physiological changes after brain stem death and management of the heart-beating donor. *Continuing Education in Anaesthesia Critical Care & Pain* 2012; 12 (5): 225–229.

19. D

Pleural fluid is classically described as either a transudate or exudate. Exudative pleural effusions meet at least one of the following criteria (Light's criteria), whereas transudative pleural effusions meet none:

(i) the ratio of pleural fluid protein to serum protein is 0.5

(ii) the ratio of pleural fluid lactic dehydrogenase (LDH) and serum LDH is 0.6

(iii) pleural fluid LDH is more than two-thirds normal upper limit for serum

This patient has an exudate according to Light's criteria. The low glucose and pH indicate this is more likely to be an empyema than pancreatitis as the cause of exudate. The others are transudates.

Paramasivam E, Bodenham A. Pleural fluid collections in critically ill patients. *Continuing Education in Anaesthesia Critical Care & Pain* 2007; 7 (1): 10–14.

20. A

Botulism should be suspected in an IV drug user. The classic signs are acute symmetrical, descending paralysis with no sensory deficit, no fever, and no lack of awareness. Guillain–Barré syndrome patients usually have a history of a febrile illness then ascending muscle weakness starting in the hands and feet with accompanying loss of sensation and pain. Patients with myasthenia or Eaton–Lambert syndrome demonstrate fatigability in skeletal muscles. This means they worsen with repetitive muscle contraction and improve with muscle resting. Viral encephalitis is associated with fever, altered mental state, and asymmetrical weakness.

Wenham T , Cohen A. Botulism. *Continuing Education in Anaesthesia Critical Care & Pain* 2008; 8 (1): 21–25.

1. **A 56-year-old woman attends the chronic pain clinic with a history of chronic pain in her right arm. What is the best way to differentiate between chronic regional pain syndrome (CRPS) type 1 and CRPS type 2?**
   A. History
   B. Clinical examination
   C. Nerve conduction studies
   D. Budapest criteria
   E. Degree of resulting physical disability

2. **A 40-year-old man is referred to the pain clinic complaining of gnawing pain in his right thigh. He is wheelchair bound following a spinal cord transection at T12 two years previously. He denies any recent injury and is systemically well. The most likely cause of his pain is:**
   A. A pathological pelvic fracture
   B. A deep venous thrombosis
   C. Psychosomatic pain
   D. Neuropathic pain following the accident
   E. Nociceptive pain following the accident

3. **You anaesthetize a 35-year-old woman for mastectomy and axillary clearance alongside your Consultant. Your Consultant suggests you include nitrous oxide in your gas mix instead of your planned oxygen/air/volatile mix. What is the best reason for using nitrous oxide in this patient?**
   A. To augment the postoperative analgesic regimen
   B. To expedite recovery from general anaesthesia
   C. To reduce the total opioid requirement
   D. To reduce the incidence of chronic scar pain developing
   E. To reduce the incidence of airway complications at induction and emergence

4. **A 64-year-old man with peripheral vascular disease requires a below knee amputation. He is taking regular paracetamol and 30 mg of morphine sulphate (MST) twice daily with Sevredol 10 mg 4 hourly for breakthrough. What would be the optimal analgesic technique to manage stump pain postoperatively and reduce his chance of developing phantom limb pain?**

    A. Intrathecal opioid
    B. An epidural running for 48 hours before surgery
    C. An infusion of IV ketamine intraoperatively
    D. A perineural sciatic nerve catheter and with a local anaesthetic infusion running for 72–96 hours
    E. Pre-medicate with pregabalin and use a morphine patient-controlled analgesia (PCA) device postoperatively

5. **A 67-year-old man with peripheral vascular disease presents as an emergency for a right above knee amputation. He is currently on clopidogrel. You administer a general anaesthetic including intravenous ketamine as part of your perioperative pain management. What is the principal site for the pharmacological action of ketamine?**

    A. GABA receptors
    B. Opioid receptors
    C. Monoaminergic receptors
    D. Cholinergic receptors
    E. NMDA receptors

6. **You anaesthetize a 38-year-old woman for mastectomy and axillary clearance. Which analgesic technique is best to reduce the incidence of chronic scar pain postoperatively?**

    A. Thoracic epidural
    B. Paravertebral block
    C. Cryo-analgesia to intercostal nerves perioperatively
    D. PCA morphine
    E. Lidocaine infusion via wound catheter

7. **A 36-year-old patient has chronic scar pain following mastectomy. She is to be given a new analgesic patch to try. Which method of delivery will maximize any placebo effect gained from the treatment?**

    A. Ask GP to prescribe and patient to apply herself
    B. Refer to practice nurse for information and first application
    C. Refer to nurse-led pain clinic session for information and first application
    D. Prescribe the most expensive brand of the patch
    E. Give patient written information detailing the efficacy of the patch in trials

8. **Which of the following methods is best used for measuring pain in a 90-year-old patient with dementia who has sustained a fractured neck of femur?**
   A. Verbal descriptor score
   B. Visual analogue score
   C. Numerical rating scale
   D. Wong–Baker faces scale
   E. Behavioural assessment

9. **Which of the following gives the most accurate description of the way each tool is used to assess pain?**
   A. The McGill Pain Questionnaire provides an objective measure of pain
   B. The McGill Pain Questionnaire measures sensory, affective, and cognitive aspects of pain
   C. The HADS (Hospital Anxiety and Depression Scale) is useful in assessing acute pain
   D. The HADS uses numerical sub-scales to assess each question
   E. The Brief Pain Inventory is most relevant to cancer pain

10. **You consent a patient for caudal epidural steroid injection on the interventional pain list. Which combination of risks best reflects what you would discuss with the patient?**
    A. Failure, infection, nerve damage, risk of dural puncture headache
    B. Failure, infection, worsening of pain afterwards, constipation
    C. Infection, worsening of pain afterwards, impotence, and urinary retention
    D. Failure, infection, worsening of pain afterwards, leg weakness post procedure
    E. Failure, infection, worsening of pain afterwards, delayed onset of any benefit

11. **Which of the following groups of characteristics describes the patient who is most likely to suffer from chronic pain?**
    A. Male, 75 years of age, retired, low educational background
    B. Female, 75 years of age, retired, high educational background
    C. Male 50 years of age, unemployed, low educational background
    D. Female, 50 years of age, unemployed, low educational background
    E. Female, 45 years of age, unemployed, high educational background

12. **A 45-year-old man presents to clinic with a diagnosis of chronic headache. Extensive investigation has found no abnormal results. He has tried a variety of drugs which have failed to help the pain. He asks about non-pharmacological therapies. Which would be the best intervention to try first?**
    A. Acupuncture
    B. Pain management programme
    C. Botulinum toxin injections
    D. Greater occipital nerve block
    E. TENS machine

13. You review a 46-year-old woman in the pain clinic. She describes a right-sided burning pain confined to the area supplied by T6 following an episode of shingles six months previously. You diagnose post-herpetic neuralgia (PHN) The best treatment to control her pain acutely is:

    A. Regular diclofenac and co-codamol
    B. Famciclovir
    C. Gabapentin
    D. Lidocaine patch
    E. Nortriptyline

14. On the acute pain round you review a 56-year-old man who had a midline laparotomy yesterday for bowel obstruction. He has a thoracic epidural running at 6 mL/hour with 0.1% levobupivacaine and 2 µg/mL fentanyl. He complains of severe abdominal pain which got much worse this morning. On examination his epidural block is to T6. The most likely reason for his pain is:

    A. The epidural has become disconnected overnight
    B. He has been asleep all night and no pain assessments have been carried out
    C. The rate of epidural infusion is too low
    D. He has suffered an anastomotic dehiscence
    E. He has a low pain threshold

15. A 24-year-old female with chronic back pain attends the chronic pain clinic seeking improvement in her pain. She reports a pain score of 9/10. She takes tramadol 100 mg four times per day, ibuprofen 400 mg three times daily, pregabalin 300 mg twice daily, and amitriptyline 25 mg daily, yet remains unable to work due to pain. What is the next best step in the management of her pain?

    A. Commence MST/sevredol
    B. Increase dose pregabalin
    C. Refer for pain physiotherapy
    D. Refer for spinal cord stimulation
    E. Refer to orthopaedic surgeons for surgery

16. Which of the following methods is best able to diagnose a neuropathic pain condition?

    A. History and examination
    B. Nerve conduction studies
    C. Electromyography
    D. Magnetic resonance imaging (MRI) scan
    E. Transient needle nerve block

17. **A 36-year-old woman presents with migrainous headaches without aura. She reports having two headaches per week, every week. The most appropriate pharmaceutical option for her is:**

    A. Regular daily NSAIDs with paracetamol when headache comes on
    B. Regular daily NSAIDs with oral triptan when headache comes on
    C. Prophylactic topiramate
    D. Prophylactic propranolol
    E. Botulinium toxin A every three months

18. **A 52-year-old female patient attends the pain clinic as an outpatient. She was diagnosed with classical trigeminal neuralgia six months previously. She was commenced on carbamazepine with incremental dose increases. Her pain is now controlled on 600 mg carbamazepine daily but she complains that the side effects of fatigue and dizziness are becoming troublesome. Which of the following is the best management option?**

    A. Reduce carbamazepine dose
    B. Stop carbamazepine, start phenytoin
    C. Stop carbamazepine, start oxycarbamazepine at increased dose
    D. Commence gabapentin concurrently
    E. Refer for surgical or interventional treatment

19. **A patient in the pain clinic is reluctant to reduce her dose of opioid. The Consultant thinks she may have opioid-induced hyperalgesia (OIH). This diagnosis is best supported by which statement below:**

    A. The dose–response curve shifts to the right
    B. The dose–response curve shifts to the left
    C. She has pain that is different to her original complaint
    D. She has been on opioids for over one year
    E. She reports increasing side effects of opioids

20. **A patient attends your pain clinic taking several drugs for mixed nociceptive and neuropathic pain. Which combination is most likely to increase the risk of serotonin syndrome?**

    A. Ondansetron, morphine, amitriptyline
    B. Nortriptyline, pregabalin, tramadol
    C. Tapentadol, pregabalin, nefopam
    D. Amitriptyline, tramadol, cyclizine
    E. Duloxetine, tramadol, paracetamol

1. A

CRPS type 2 requires a history of specific nerve injury for diagnosis. CRPS type 1 may look and feel the same on clinical examination but can occur following any type of injury in the affected area.

Nerve conduction studies primarily test thick myelinated Aα and B fibres in mixed peripheral nerves. They do not test small Ad and C fibres primarily affected in chronic pain.

The Budapest criteria must be met for diagnosis of both types of CRPS but cannot differentiate between the two. The degree of physical impairment is important in the ongoing management of such patients but is not part of the diagnostic criteria for either condition.

Ganty P, Chawla R. Complex regional pain syndrome: recent updates. *Continuing Education in Anaesthesia Critical Care & Pain* 2014; 14 (2): 79–84.

2. D

Neuropathic pain is extremely common in those with spinal cord injury. It is estimated to affect 70% of this group. It is thought to be due to sprouting of new nerve fibres below the level of spinal cord lesion. While essential for recovery, these neurones are hyperexcitable and their responses not always positive.

There is no history to suggest a pelvic fracture nor metastatic disease. Psychosomatic implies no organic cause of pain but this patient has definite underlying causes. However, psychological issues can arise from pain and input from psychology is very helpful in managing pain.

Nociceptive pain should not persist past 12 weeks.

Hadjipavlou G, Cortese AM, Ramaswamy B. Spinal cord injury and chronic pain. *BJA Education* 2016; 16 (8): 264–268.

3. D

Mastectomy is complicated by a high incidence of postoperative chronic pain including scar pain. This is due to many factors but an important method of prevention is good intraoperative analgesia including use of nitrous oxide as an adjunct.

Nitrous oxide has fallen out of favour in recent years with trends towards using a 'cleaner' gas mix of oxygen/air/volatile to reduce postoperative nausea and vomiting. This must be balanced against the high incidence of chronic pain following this procedure particularly affecting younger female patients.

Australian and New Zealand College of Anaesthetists and Faculty of Pain Medicine. *Acute Pain Management: Scientific Evidence*, 4th Edition 2015.

4. D

It is important to treat acute pain effectively with good quality analgesia. This reduces both the pathophysiological stress response and the patient's psychological contribution. Poor analgesia in the immediate postoperative period predisposes to reduced functional recovery and the development of chronic stump and phantom limb pain.

Prolonged analgesia via continuous perineural blockade is the gold standard analgesic technique for early management of stump and phantom pain. It should be extended beyond 72 hours wherever possible. It is safe, effective, opioid sparing with few side effects, and requires low levels of monitoring. The other options are all used, either alone or in combination, and provide reasonable analgesia. Each has its own merits and side effect profile.

Studies of epidural analgesia have been disappointing. They have failed to show any reduction in the incidence of chronic pain or phantom pain post amputation but in most studies the infusion was stopped early after operation. Aside from this they have a 10% failure rate, a risk of infection and other morbidities in an often diabetic or anticoagulated patient group.

Neil MJE. Pain after amputation. *BJA Education* 2016; 16 (3): 107–112.

5. E

The principal action of ketamine is non-competitive antagonism of the NMDA receptor. It also interacts with all the other receptors mentioned. Perioperative ketamine has been shown to reduce the incidence of persistent post-surgical pain.

Tsui PY, Chu MC. Ketamine: An old drug revitalized in pain medicine *BJA Education* 2017; 17 (3): 84–87.

6. B

The intensity of acute pain is a consistent predictor of post-surgical chronic pain (PSCP). PSCP is most common in areas where nerves are damaged during surgery and those which are richly innervated (e.g. chest wall).

Paravertebral block has been shown to be effective in minimizing chronic scar pain. A thoracic epidural may also help but would confer more risks for similar benefits in mastectomy.

Identifying intercostals nerves to preserve them may help (though not mentioned in the answer) but cryo-analgesia at the time of surgery makes subsequent chronic pain worse.

PCA morphine and lidocaine wound infusion work well in the acute phase of postoperative pain but have no impact on the development of chronic pain.

Lidocaine does however reduce the incidence of PSCP but only when given intravenously.

Humble SR, Dalton AJ, Li L. A systematic review of therapeutic interventions to reduce acute and chronic post-surgical pain after amputation, thoracotomy or mastectomy. *European Journal of Pain* 2015; 19: 451–465.

7. C

Placebo effect is common and occurs in addition to the therapeutic effects of intervention. It is largely contextual and therefore is maximized when given by more senior members of staff in more specialized areas. The actual treatment given is less important than the therapeutic encounter, its rituals, symbols, and interactions which surround the application or use. Branded medicines have a larger placebo effect than generic versions, injections have a greater effect than tablets, and administration by a doctor confers more placebo effect than when given by a nurse.

Kaptchuk TJ, Miller FG. Placebo effects in medicine. *New England Journal of Medicine* 2015; 373: 8–9.

8. E

Acute pain can be assessed by any unidirectional method but options A, B, C, and D require intact cognition to understand the questions asked, the details of the scale, and to know how to respond.

Behavioural assessment is the most useful: observing facial expression, movement, or lack thereof, and the response to same. Be aware that this type of assessment, proxy reporting of pain, is less accurate than personal (self) reporting of pain by the patient and usually underestimates the amount of pain actually being experienced by the patient. It does not take into account the affective and cognitive aspects of pain which cause distress too. Communication barriers may be due to dementia or confusion and when cognition is intact but the patient is dysphasic or aphasic.

Breivik H, Borchgrevink PC, Allen SM, et al. Assessment of pain. *British Journal of Anaesthesia* 2008; 101 (1): 17–24.

Herr KA, Garand L. Assessment and measurement of pain in older adults. *Clinics in Geriatric Medicine* 2001; 17 (3): 457–478, vi.

9. B

To assess pain it is necessary to consider the affective and cognitive aspects of pain, as well as the more obvious sensory aspects. There is no objective measure of pain.

The HADS score, though useful in the overall assessment of pain as described above, does not assess the sensory aspect most relevant in acute pain. The Brief Pain Inventory was developed to assess cancer pain but is now thoroughly validated for use in persistent pain from any source or cause.

Schofield P. 'It's your age': The assessment and management of pain in older adults. *Continuing Education in Anaesthesia Critical Care & Pain* 2010; 10 (3): 93–95.

10. E

The patient must be informed of the risks of failure of the block (both technical and clinical), and infection. Nerve damage should be mentioned in context showing its rarity. Interventions in chronic pain can make the patient's pain worse in the acute phase. This is due to the needle causing additional trauma in a painful area. It should settle after five to seven days. The dura and cerebrospinal fluid end around S2 so are unlikely to be breached during caudal catheter placement.

Constipation, urinary retention, and impotence are all side effects of lumbar sympathectomy and are not relevant to caudal injections.

Collighan N, Gupta S. A epidural steroids. *Continuing Education in Anaesthesia Critical Care & Pain* 2010; 10 (1): 1–5.

11. D

There are specific risk factors for developing chronic pain. These include being female, being of a younger age (chronic pain is much reduced in the elderly), being unemployed, and being from a low educational background. Answer D contains four risk factors. No other option contains more than 2.

Feizerfan A, Sheh G. Transition from acute to chronic pain. *Continuing Education in Anaesthesia Critical Care & Pain* 2015; 15 (2): 98–102.

12. A

When considering interventions, it is important to consider the degree of invasiveness, the associated risks, and the evidence for potential benefit. Acupuncture is minimally invasive and there is some evidence of its efficacy in treating chronic headache (and low back pain). Greater occipital nerve blocks are no longer recommended as there is little evidence supporting their efficacy. Repeat blocks also introduce risks of infection, nerve damage, and increase the patient's lifetime steroid load. Botulinum toxin is considered an effective treatment and may be considered.

It is more invasive than acupuncture. A Pain management programme may be beneficial when all treatment options have been exhausted. A TENS machine could be used by the patient but there is no evidence it improves pain.

Botulinum toxin type A for the prevention of headaches in adults with chronic migraine. NICE Guideline. Available at: https://www.nice.org.uk/guidance/ta260

Linde K, Allais G, Brinkhaus B, Fei Y, et al. Acupuncture for tension type headache. April 2016 Cochrane review: Available at: http://www.cochrane.org/CD007587/SYMPT_acupuncture-tension-type-headache

13. C

PHN is a self-limiting condition and management is directed at controlling the pain while waiting for the condition to resolve itself. A multimodal approach to the analgesic regimen will provide additive effects though efficacy will vary between individuals.

Lidocaine patches work well but the effect is transient, lasting only 4–12 hours. The analgesic effect of nortriptyline and other tricyclic antidepressants is very slow and a trial of around three months is required to determine whether there is any benefit.

Gabapentin is effective and works quickly. It is also effective in treating the sleep disturbance that commonly co-exists so would be the first line therapy in this case. Opioids, while not mentioned here are only occasionally indicated for cases with extreme pain.

Paracetamol and NSAIDs alone have not been shown to be effective in PHN although they may be included as part of a multimodal approach. Famciclovir is an antiviral drug which, if given at the start of the episode of shingles, reduces the incidence of chronic pain developing after it has resolved.

Anaesthesia UK. Management of Post Herpetic Neuralgia. 2005. Available at: http://www.frca.co.uk/article.aspx?articleid=100531

14. D

Acute pain has complex aetiology and is highly variable between individuals. Pain is always subjective and the severity is, as the patient states. The rate of the epidural infusion is on the low side but on testing, his block is adequate to cover the wound. Regular pain assessment improves acute pain control but is not necessary overnight if the patient is sleeping. This would be more relevant if the epidural was a patient-controlled bolus system.

The history of any pain is always of fundamental importance including its onset, spread, character, and associated features. Complaints of pain despite a seemingly adequate spread of epidural analgesia should always be taken seriously. The patient gives a recent history of acutely worsening pain over a short period which suggests something has happened around that time, such as an intra-abdominal catastrophe.

Australia and New Zealand College of Anaesthetists and Faculty of Pain Medicine (ANZA). Acute Pain Management: Scientific Evidence (4th edition) 2015.

15. C

Pain physiotherapy would be the next best thing to offer this patient. This requires engagement from the patient. Pain psychology may have a beneficial role here too.

A short course of strong opioids may be helpful to facilitate participation in pain physiotherapy but there is no evidence for their use in the long term. Any opioid trial should be finite with no dose escalation. Opioids can lead to addiction and dependence and have many side effects. This patient is already on a large dose of tramadol and the maximum dose (600 mg daily) of pregabalin.

Spinal cord stimulation is not indicated for chronic back pain.

NICE Guideline 59: Low back pain and sciatica in over 16s: Assessment and management. Nov 2016. Available at: https://www.nice.org.uk/guidance/ng59

Chaparro L, Furlan AD, Deshpande A. The Cochrane Review: Opioids for the treatment of chronic low-back pain. Available at: http://www.cochrane.org/CD004959/BACK_opioids-for-the-treatment-of-chronic-low-back-pain

16. A

Chronic pain of any origin is best assessed with a detailed history and examination. Sometimes further investigations MAY be requested, for example a CT scan to investigate central causes such as stroke or an MRI to confirm specific nerve root compression.

E-pain Module 07 Diagnosis and Management of Neuropathic Pain. Available at: http://portal.elfh.org.uk/myElearning/Index?HierarchyId=0_196_196&programmeId=196

17. D

The patient has eight headaches per month and prophylactic treatment is indicated when a sufferer has 15 or more each month, or has a poor response to acute treatment. Both topiramate and propranolol are indicated for prophylaxis. Topiramate is teratogenic and should be used cautiously in woman of childbearing age. It can also reduce the effectiveness of hormonal contraception. Therefore, Propanolol would be a safer first-line prophylactic treatment, as would a course of acupuncture, although this was not an option here.

Botulinum toxin A is indicated for chronic migraine only (headaches more than 15 times per month).

NSAIDs, paracetamol, and triptans (oral and intranasal) are first-line acute treatments. If these fail, parenteral metoclopramide or prochlorperazine is recommended.

Poply K, Bahra A, Mehta V. Migraine. *BJA Education* 2016; 16 (11): 357–361.

Headaches in over 12s: Diagnosis and Management. NICE Clinical guideline 150, 2015. Available at: https://www.nice.org.uk/guidance/cg150

18. C

Effective treatment of trigeminal neuralgia means balancing good analgesia with minimal side effects. Several drug regimens may need to be trialled before one which suits each individual patient is found.

Carbamazepine is first-line treatment and is the most effective in treating the pain. Reducing the dose will reduce the side effects but results in unsatisfactory levels of analgesia. Changing to oxycarbamazine, a derivative of carbamazepine, is a good option; although higher doses are required for analgesia there are fewer associated side effects.

Changing to phenytoin may be required in due course but phenytoin has similarly severe side effects and no better analgesia than carbamazepine. Caution is required; carbamazepine should be slowly reduced then stopped and phenytoin gradually introduced and increased over a period of several weeks.

Gabapentin can be used concurrently with carbamazepine but there is no specific evidence of its efficacy in trigeminal neuralgia specifically.

There are several pharmacological options to be explored before considering surgical intervention.

Vasappa CK, Kapur S, Krovvidi H. Trigeminal neuralgia. *British Journal of Anaesthesia Education* 2016; 16. 10: 353.

Zakrzewska JM, Linskey ME. Trigeminal neuralgia. *British Medical Journal Clinical Evidence* 2014; 10: 1207.

19. C

OIH is a real and challenging clinical situation. It must be differentiated from tolerance (where the patient reports the same type of pain but of increased intensity), and disease progression (when the pain may spread to new areas). OIH causes increased sensitivity to painful stimuli and the pain has different characteristics to the original pain being treated with opioids. OIH can occur during short periods of treatment with opioids including acute use in the perioperative period.

Velayudhan A, Bellingham G, Morley-Forster P. Opioid-induced hyperalgesia. *Continuing Education in Anaesthesia, Critical Care & Pain* 2014; 14 (3): 125–129.

20. B

Serotonin syndrome is a rare complication of medicines which act by inhibiting reuptake of serotonin and increasing the free drug concentration. Its onset can be gradual and easily missed in the early stages. Patients with polypharmacy should have their medicines reviewed regularly and be asked specifically about side effects.

All three drugs in answer B have an element of serotonin reuptake inhibition and tramadol especially in this regard. All other options only contain two drugs working in this way. All antidepressants have an effect on serotonin levels, as do tramadol and tapentadol. Nefopam is an analgesic of as yet unknown mechanism of action but is not believed to work via opioid or 5HT receptors. Paracetamol, cyclizine, and ondansetron do not increase the risk of serotonin syndrome.

Lamberg JJ, Gordon VN. Serotonin syndrome in a patient with chronic pain polypharmacy. *Pain Medicine* 2014; 15: 1429–1435.

1. **A patient is taking 60 mg of dihydrocodeine four times per day for neuropathic leg pain. He had planned to reduce his usage but quickly stopped when he developed diarrhoea and shaking when he first missed a dose. He is reluctant to try again as fears his pain will become worse. What best describes the patients state with regard to opioids?**
    A. He is addicted
    B. He is dependent
    C. He has developed tolerance
    D. He has withdrawal
    E. He has adverse reactions

2. **Which of the following operations carries the weakest indication for paravertebral block?**
    A. Mastectomy and axillary clearance
    B. Lateral thoracotomy
    C. Open cholecystectomy
    D. Midline laparotomy
    E. Inguinal hernia repair

3. **Regarding mechanical circulatory support with an intra-aortic balloon pump. The best choice of gas for balloon inflation is:**
    A. Hydrogen
    B. Helium
    C. Oxygen
    D. Nitrogen
    E. Carbon dioxide

4. **Regarding the description of a skewed dataset, the most commonly quoted measure of data spread is:**
    A. Interquartile range
    B. Standard deviation
    C. Range
    D. Standard error of the mean
    E. Variance

5. **You anaesthetize a patient for laser vocal cord surgery. The patient is ventilated via a laser tube with an oxygen/air/desflurane mix. A fire is ignited in the airway. What should your immediate action be?**

   A. Remove the endotracheal tube

   B. Flood the operative site with saline

   C. Switch off the anaesthetic machine

   D. Disconnect the breathing circuit

   E. Reduce FiO_2 to 21%

6. **The use of mannitol as an osmotic diuretic is recommended as a standard of care by consensus guidance during management of which condition below?**

   A. Renal protection in cardiac surgery

   B. Renal protection in non-cardiac vascular surgery

   C. Renal transplantation

   D. Intracranial pressure

   E. Rhabdomyolysis

7. **An 82-year-old woman presents with fractured neck of femur. Her past medical history includes transient ischaemic attack, hypertension, and stage 4 breast cancer. Her medication includes bisoprolol, bendroflumethiazide, and clopidogrel. She lives alone and is usually able to climb two flights of stairs. Her blood tests are unremarkable and resting electrocardiogram (ECG) is normal. The FY1 has noted a cardiac murmur on examination. What is the most appropriate next step?**

   A. Postpone surgery pending echocardiography

   B. Because of terminal diagnosis, cancel surgery, and refer to palliative care

   C. Stop clopidogrel for seven days and then proceed under spinal anaesthesia

   D. Arrange a platelet transfusion and proceed under general anaesthesia (GA)

   E. Proceed under GA

8. **You review a 67-year-old man at the pre-assessment clinic. He has been smoking 20 cigarettes a day for more than 40 years. He has a chronic cough and is short of breath on exertion. You order pulmonary function tests to investigate further. Which of the following would best support a diagnosis of moderate chronic obstructive pulmonary disease (COPD)?**

   A. Forced expiratory volume in 1 second (FEV_1) 81% predicted

   B. Increased gas transfer coefficient

   C. FEV_1:FVC (forced vital capacity) ratio post bronchodilator of 0.6

   D. Increased vital capacity

   E. Decreased carbon monoxide transfer factor

9. **When reviewing a 57-year-old lady on the daily intensive care unit (ICU) round you notice she is grimacing, her upper limbs are fully flexed, and she is coughing on her ET tube after turning and dressing changes. She was admitted 24 hours ago following an emergency laparotomy for a perforated duodenal ulcer. She is currently on propofol and morphine infusions. What would be the best management of this patient?**
   A. Add an infusion of atracurium
   B. Change to midazolam sedation
   C. Increase the morphine infusion
   D. Add a regular NSAID
   E. Increase the propofol infusion

10. **You are required to anaesthetize a 29-year-old para 1 at term for category 2 caesarean section due to failure to progress in labour. She is using remifentanil patient-controlled analgesia (PCA) for analgesia. She had a normal vaginal delivery previously. She has congenital bicuspid aortic valve and the gradient across the valve is 25 mmHg. The best anaesthetic for caesarean section is:**
    A. *De novo* epidural and top up
    B. Spinal
    C. Combined spinal/epidural
    D. GA using rapid sequence induction
    E. GA using target-controlled infusion (TCI) propofol and remifentanil

11. **A 69-year-old man is scheduled for a coronary artery bypass graft. He past medical history includes ischaemic heart disease, type 2 diabetes, and hypercholesterolaemia. He is concerned about the risks of his surgery. What is the most common significant neurological complication following this surgery?**
    A. Transient ischaemic attack
    B. Raised intracranial pressure
    C. Intracranial haemorrhage
    D. Postoperative cognitive dysfunction (POCD)
    E. Ischaemic stroke

12. **A patient in the High Dependency Unit requires renal replacement therapy (RRT). The patient has no central intravenous access at present. What is the preferred site for a renal replacement line?**
    A. Left subclavian vein
    B. Right internal jugular vein
    C. Right femoral vein
    D. Left internal jugular vein
    E. Right subclavian vein

13. **You have admitted a woman to ICU with a body mass index of 16 and a very poor nutritional state. You start controlled nasogastric feeding with a standard bag, noting that she is at high risk of refeeding syndrome. What is the most important additional compound to replace?**
   A. Thiamine
   B. Vitamin B12
   C. Folate
   D. Vitamin D
   E. Glutamine

14. **A healthy 28-year-old lady had a normal spontaneous vaginal delivery (SVD) two days ago. She had an epidural for labour which was sited without complication. She is now complaining of a constant band-like headache and is intolerant of noise. She has no other neurological signs or symptoms. What is the most likely cause of her headache?**
   A. Pre-eclampsia
   B. Cortical vein thrombosis
   C. Post-dural puncture headache
   D. Tension headache
   E. Meningitis

15. **When considering statistical test, which of the following best describes the analysis of variance (ANOVA) test?**
   A. A test to compare two normally distributed independent groups
   B. A test to compare two normally distributed matched groups
   C. A test that compares the mean of one sample group against a known value
   D. A test that compares greater than three sample proportions of categorical data
   E. A test that compares three or more normally distributed groups of interval data

16. **A 27-year-old woman presents with acute breathlessness and respiratory failure. She has signs of a current chest infection. She has a background history of worsening exercise tolerance over the previous three months. She improves with rest and has no muscle pain. On examination she has generalized muscle fatigability, ptosis, and diplopia. She has normal reflexes, sensation, and coordination. An appropriate treatment includes:**
   A. Atropine
   B. Edrophonium
   C. Neostigmine
   D. Hydrocotrisone
   E. Pyridostigmine

17. An obstetric patient with severe pre-eclampsia is managed in labour ward high dependency. You plan to site a radial arterial line for monitoring and blood sampling. The midwife asks how to prime the arterial line set. What is the recommended flush solution?

A. Hartmann's solution

B. Glucose 5%

C. Glucose 10%

D. Saline 0.9%

E. Saline 0.45%

18. A male adult patient is in intensive care for 26 days and is recovering from sepsis. He has had multiple central lines during this admission. He has deteriorated with a new septic episode. He now requires a central line for vasopressor therapy. A left subclavian site is chosen as the most favourable. The most appropriate central line is:

A. Tunnelled catheter, three lumens, 20 cm long

B. Tunnelled catheter, three lumens, 25 cm long

C. Non-tunnelled catheter, single lumen, 20 cm

D. Non-tunnelled catheter, triple lumen, 20 cm

E. Non-tunnelled catheter, triple lumen, 25 cm

19. A 26-year-old primiparous patient requires a category one caesarean section for prolonged fetal bradycardia. Which drug combination provides the best intubating conditions, assuming appropriate doses of each are used?

A. Propofol, alfentanil, rocuronium

B. Propofol, suxamethonium

C. Thiopentone, rocuronium

D. Thiopentone, suxamethonium

E. TCI propofol and remifentanil

20. A 54-year-old patient has undergone brainstem death testing and is confirmed brainstem dead. He is on a voluntary organ donation register but his relatives are not willing for organ donation. How should you proceed?

A. Check the patient's human leukocyte antigen (HLA) status

B. Mobilize the organ retrieval team

C. Respect the patient's wishes

D. Respect the relatives' wishes

E. Seek the coroner's decision over the telephone

21. **You are reviewing a 26-year-old para 1 + 0 woman on the postnatal ward. The evening before she had delivered a live baby boy of 3.9 kg by mid-cavity forceps. In labour, an epidural had been sited but had not worked well so was not topped up for delivery. Instead, in theatre a spinal was performed without complication. The woman has no complaints but mentions she noticed the front and side of her left thigh felt numb while washing in the shower. On examination there is no motor deficit nor any red flag signs of spinal cord injury. The most likely cause of the numbness is:**

A. Residual effect from epidural local anaesthetic

B. Pre-existing prolapsed vertebral disc at L2,3

C. Psychosomatic as does not reflect any dermatomal distribution

D. Fetal head compressing lumbosacral trunk

E. Prolonged lithotomy position

22. **A 60-year-old man with obstructive sleep apnoea (OSA) and atrial fibrillation (AF) presents for elective hernia repair. He takes warfarin and his INR is currently 1.5. What is the best anaesthetic management?**

A. Controlled ventilation, desflurane, remifentanil infusion, and an inguinal field bloc

B. Controlled ventilation sevoflurane, remifentanil, and an inguinal field block

C. Spontaneous ventilation, propofol TCI, remifentanil infusion, and inguinal field block

D. Spontaneous ventilation, sevoflurane, and inguinal field block

E. Spontaneous ventilation, propofol TCI, PCA morphine

23. **You anaesthetize a 40-year-old 70-kg man using isoflurane to maintain anaesthesia and a circle system. The vaporizer dial setting is 2.0%, the end-tidal isoflurane concentration 1.2% and the fresh gas flow (FGF) through the vaporizer is 400 mL/min of an oxygen/air mixture. Which of the following is the fastest method of increasing the depth of anaesthesia?**

A. Increase the vaporizer setting to isoflurane 2.5%

B. Increase the FGF to 8 L/min

C. Change to sevoflurane

D. Switch to a nitrous oxide/oxygen mix with $FiO_2 = 0.3$

E. Switch to a nitrous oxide/oxygen mix with $FiO_2 = 0.5$

24. **A 7-year-old boy with significant snoring attends for day case tonsillectomy. He is otherwise well. Which of the following would preclude him being discharged home postoperatively?**

A. Having NSAIDs in theatre

B. Having 7 mg of morphine perioperatively

C. His parents are both heavy smokers

D. His parents do not have a car

E. He has spat out a few blood streaked secretions postoperatively

25. **You prescribe a fentanyl patch for a patient in the chronic pain clinic. Which physicochemical feature of drugs most improves their efficacy via the transdermal route?**
    A. Low molecular weight
    B. Low lipid solubility
    C. Low pKa
    D. Melting point above 37°C
    E. Active metabolites

26. **According to accepted receptor theory, a partial agonist**
    A. Has reduced receptor affinity when compared with a full agonist
    B. Produces a concentration–effect curve similar to a full agonist but will take longer to attain maximum activity levels
    C. Produces the same level of response as that achieved by a full agonist in the presence of a competitive antagonist
    D. Is less potent than a full agonist
    E. Can bind to both agonist and antagonist binding sites

27. **Regarding pharmacokinetics in the elderly**
    A. Bioavailability of many drugs is increased
    B. Phase 2 metabolic reactions in liver are significantly reduced
    C. The volume of distribution for water soluble drugs is increased
    D. The duration of action of fat soluble drugs is reduced
    E. eGFR is unchanged

28. **You assess a 23-year-old woman for consideration of labour epidural analgesia. She is a 40/52 gestation primigravida in established labour with no significant medical history. While in the room the midwife expresses concerns regarding the cardiotocograph (CTG) and asks the senior midwife to attend. Which of the following is most indicative of a pathological CTG?**
    A. Baseline rate of 140 bpm with early decelerations
    B. Baseline rate of 135 bpm with late decelerations
    C. Baseline rate of 135 bpm with persistently absent variability
    D. Baseline rate of 120 bpm with normal variability
    E. Baseline rate of 140 bpm with transient accelerations

29. **A 69-year-old woman was admitted to ICU 24 hours ago following a catastrophic intracerebral bleed. There was no possible neurosurgical intervention. Her past medical history includes hypertension and hypothyroidism. She is a non-smoker. She remains GCS 3 and you and your consultant are about to perform brainstem death testing to diagnose death using neurological criteria. Which of the following most correctly describes the $PaCO_2$ criteria necessary for apnoea testing?**

    A. $PaCO_2$ of 4–5.3 kPa prior to commencing test and then a rise of ≥1 kPa at end of test
    B. $PaCO_2$ of 4–4.5 kPa prior to commencing apnoea test and then a rise of ≥0.5 kPa at end of test
    C. $PaCO_2$ of ≥6 kPa prior to testing with a rise of ≥0.5 kPa at end of test
    D. $PaCO_2$ of 4.5–5.3 kPa prior to commencing test with a rise of ≥2 kPa
    E. $PaCO_2$ of ≥6.5 kPa prior to commencing test with a rise of ≥0.5 kPa at end of test

30. **A 54-year-old man is listed for an amputation of his left big toe. He has chronic renal impairment, stable angina, heart failure (NYHA grade 2) and type 2 diabetes. On reviewing his blood results and ECG from this morning you discover his potassium is 7.3 mmol/L and his ECG shows 52 bpm sinus rhythm with flattening of P waves and tall T waves. What would be the best initial treatment?**

    A. 10 units of Actrapid in 50 mL 50% dextrose over 15 minutes intravenously
    B. Nebulized salbutamol 5 mg
    C. Oral calcium resonium
    D. Bolus of calcium gluconate 10% 10 mL intravenously
    E. Commence haemodialysis

1. B

Dependence can be both psychological and physical. Psychological dependence is characterized by fear of stopping drugs and physical dependence by the appearance of withdrawal effects when the drug is stopped. D is correct (withdrawal), and it could also be said that he is suffering an adverse reaction (E), but B is the better, complete answer.

Addiction is characterized by compulsive drug seeking behaviour and ingestion despite clear evidence of the substance causing ongoing harm. Tolerance occurs when the patient requires higher doses of opioid to achieve the same effect.

Tordoff SG, Ganty P. Chronic pain and prescription opioid misuse. *Continuing Education in Anaesthesia Critical Care & Pain* 2010; 10 (5): 158–161.

2. D

Paravertebral block has been described and may be indicated for unilateral surgical procedures in the thoracoabdominal region. All of these operations are unilateral except for the midline laparotomy.

Tighe SQM, Greene MD, Rajadurai N. Paravertebral block. *Continuing Education in Anaesthesia, Critical Care & Pain* 2010; 10 (5) 133–137.

3. B

Significant volumes of gas (25–50 mL) have to be moved in and out of the aortic balloon in very short periods of time. Helium is therefore the best choice because its viscosity/density is low compared with other gases which might be used and allows rapid passage through a narrow femoral catheter. Additionally, in the event of balloon rupture *in situ*, helium is easily absorbed and would therefore be removed from bubbles in the circulation faster than other more insoluble gases.

Krishna M, Zacharowski K. Principles of intra-aortic balloon pump counterpulsation. *Continuing Education in Anaesthesia, Critical Care & Pain* 2009; 9 (1): 24–28.

4. A

The interquartile range (IQR) is often quoted when referring to interval data that is not normally distributed. Additionally, it is frequently represented graphically together with the median value as a boxplot or box and whisker diagram.

McCluskey A, Lalkhen AG. Statistics II: Central tendency and spread of data. *Continuing Education in Anaesthesia, Critical Care & Pain* 2007; 7 (4): 127–130.

5. B

Fires are a very real risk during laser airway surgery since all the requirements for fire are present: oxygen, fuel (airway devices), and energy ignition (laser). Should a fire ignite in the airway, the surgeon and anaesthetist must immediately switch off the laser and flood the operation site with saline. Following this, the anaesthetic breathing system should be disconnected temporarily. There should be consideration of removing the endotracheal tube as even laser tubes can be ignited. In this scenario, the patient should then be ventilated with air using a face mask and separate breathing system.

Kitching AJ, Edge CJ. Lasers and surgery. *BJA CEPD Reviews* 2003; 8 (5): 143–146.

6. D

Mannitol is a standard of care for the management of intracranial hypertension and is recommended by consensus guidelines. There is little evidence to support its continued use for other indications, such as renal protection during cardiac and vascular surgery, or for prophylaxis against acute renal failure in rhabdomyolysis. Following renal transplantation, adequate hydration alone appears to be effective.

Shawkat H, Westwood M, Mortimer A. Mannitol: a review of its clinical uses. *Continuing Education in Anaesthesia, Critical Care & Pain* 2012; 12 (2): 82–85.

7. E

By way of formal risk assessment, this patient's Nottingham Hip Fracture (NHF) score is 5/10 which predicts mortality of around 10% at 30 days. When a hip fracture complicates a terminal illness, the multidisciplinary team should still consider the role of surgery as part of a palliative care approach to minimize pain. Surgery is the best treatment of acute pain in all hip fracture patients. While her life expectancy is certainly limited, living at home unaided suggests death from metastases is not imminent enough to subject her to the pain and problematic nursing involved with an unfixed hip fracture. Most hip fracture patients should be treated in a fast track pathway with surgery on the day of, or the day after admission. Correctable comorbidities should be identified and treated immediately so that surgery is not delayed. Surgery should not be postponed to stop clopidogrel, nor for platelets to be administered prophylactically. Marginally greater blood loss should be expected. Echocardiography is controversial in the patient with a murmur. In the context of normal ECG, reasonable exercise tolerance and absence of significant other symptoms such as angina or syncope in this patient, the majority of anaesthetists are likely to proceed without delay for echocardiography.

Griffiths R, Alper J, Beckingsale A, et al. Association of Anaesthetists of Great Britain and Ireland. Management of proximal femoral fractures 2011. *Anaesthesia* 2012; 67: 85–98.

Maxwell L, White S. Anaesthetic management of patients with hip fractures: An update. *Continuing Education in Anaesthesia Critical Care & Pain* 2013; 13 (5): 179–183.

Management of hip fractures in adults. NICE Guideline 124. Available at: https://www.nice.org.uk/guidance/cg124/chapter/Recommendations

8. C

The NICE guidelines exist to help the diagnosis and assessment of COPD. Anyone over 35 who smokes and has symptoms including cough, exertional breathlessness, and excess sputum production should be investigated primarily using spirometry. A FEV_1/FVC ratio post bronchodilator of <0.7 would be diagnostic of COPD. FEV_1% predicted useful for severity grading.

FEV_1/FVC ratio <0.7 and FEV_1% predicted >80% – mild COPD or stage 1

FEV_1/FVC ratio <0.7 and FEV_1% predicted 50–79% –moderate COPD or stage 2

FEV_1/FVC ratio <0.7 and FEV_1% predicted 30–49% – severe COPD or stage 3

FEV_1/FVC ratio <0.7 and FEV_1% predicted <30% – very severe COPD or stage 4

In COPD, the vital capacity, the carbon monoxide transfer factor, and the gas transfer coefficient are all reduced.

Lumb A, Biercamp C. Chronic obstructive pulmonary disease and anaesthesia. *Continuing Education in Anaesthesia Critical Care & Pain* 2014; 14 (1): 1–5.

9. C

The issue here is pain rather than problems with sedation or ventilation. Grimacing, flexion of limbs, muscle tension, and compliance with ventilation have a high specificity and sensitivity for predicting significant pain in postoperative ICU patients exposed to a painful procedure. When a patient is unable to communicate the Critical Care Pain Observation Tool or Behavioural Pain Scale scoring systems should be used which look at the factors mentioned above.

NSAIDS would be contraindicated in this case.

Treatment of pain in ICU should be multi-modal but is usually best managed by iv administration. This associated with fast onset and is easiest to titrate to effect.

Narayanan M, Venkataraju A, Jennings J. Analgesia in intensive care: Part 1. *BJA Education* 2016; 16 (2) 72–78.

10. C

This represents mild to moderate aortic stenosis which is well tolerated in pregnancy. The aim of any intervention is to avoid reduction in systemic vascular resistance and maintain normal sinus rhythm.

The conduct of anaesthesia is more important than the choice of technique. Previously GA was always advocated to avoid large drops in SVR and myocardial contractility resulting from regional sympathetic blocks to T4; however, in the last decade, reports show carefully managed and controlled spinal and epidural anaesthesia is increasingly used. This patient has tolerated a term pregnancy and delivery before. There is time for a regional technique to be performed but perhaps not for a *de novo* epidural to be established. A combined spinal epidural (CSE) will allow more rapid onset of block whilst avoiding the cardiovascular changes associated with a full dose single shot spinal. Uterine displacement must be maintained throughout to avoid reduction in venous return and filling pressure. Heart rate should be maintained (fixed stroke volume means any reduction in HR will reduce cardiac output). Oxytocin bolus should be avoided, an infusion is preferable to avoid tachycardia and hypotension. Consider arterial line placement perioperatively.

Brown J, Morgan-Hughes N. Aortic stenosis and non-cardiac surgery. *Continuing Education in Anaesthesia Critical Care and Pain Medicine* 2005; 5 (1): 1–4.

11. D

POCD is the most common complication with short term cognitive decline occurring in 20–50% of patients. Long-term POCD lasting greater than six months occurs in 10–30% patients.

Tan AMY, Amoako D. Postoperative cognitive dysfunction after cardiac surgery. *Continuing Education in Anaesthesia Critical Care & Pain* 2013; 13 (6): 218–223.

12. B

KDIGO Clinical Practice guideline for acute kidney injury listed the right internal jugular site as the first choice for vascular access catheters. The subclavian is the least preferred because of higher rate of stenosis formation with chronic use. The femoral vein would be the second choice. The right internal jugular should be used in preference to the left because it allows improved delivery of RRT with a straighter anatomical course.

Hall NA, Fox AJ. Renal replacement therapies in critical care. *Continuing Education in Anaesthesia Critical Care & Pain*, 2006; 6 (5) 197–202.

13. A

It is extremely important to replace thiamine (as intravenous Pabrinex) when it is likely to be deficient in order to prevent neurological complications. Thiamine is not usually found in standard enteral feed.

Macdonald K, Page K, Brown L, Bryden D. Parenteral nutrition in critical care. *Continuing Education in Anaesthesia Critical Care & Pain* 2013; 13 (1): 1–5.

See also ESPEN and NICE guidelines on enteral and parenteral nutrition.

14. D

Tension headache is the commonest cause of post-partum headache often due to hormone level fluctuation, sleep deprivation, dehydration, and caffeine withdrawal. It is characterized by a band-like headache and is usually self-limiting. There are no other signs or symptoms in the question to suggest a more sinister cause.

Sabharwal A, Stocks GM. Postpartum headache: diagnosis and management. *Continuing Education in Anaesthesia Critical Care & Pain* 2011; 11 (5): 181–185.

15. E

    A describes the un-paired Student's t-test
    B describes a paired Student's t-test
    C describes a Wilcoxon rank sum test for non-normally distributed data or a one sample t-test for normally distributed data
    D describes a chi-squared test
    E describes ANOVA

McCluskey A, Lalkhen AG. Statistics III: Probability and statistical tests. *Continuing Education in Anaesthesia Critical Care & Pain* 2007; 7 (5): 167–170.

16. B

The patient has myasthenia gravis (MG). This has a female preponderance. MG is an autoimmune disease characterized by weakness and fatigability of skeletal muscles, with improvement following rest. It may be localized to specific muscle groups or more generalized. MG is caused by a decrease in the numbers of postsynaptic acetylcholine receptors at the neuromuscular junction, which decreases the capacity of the neuromuscular endplate to transmit the nerve signal. Deterioration can be precipitated by infection as in this case. Myasthenic crisis and cholinergic crisis can present in similar ways. This patient has no diagnosis nor medication. The Tensilon (edrophonium) challenge test is useful in diagnosing MG and in distinguishing myasthenic crisis from cholinergic crisis. A positive response is not completely specific for MG because several other conditions (e.g. amyotrophic lateral sclerosis) may also respond to edrophonium with increased strength. Patients who respond generally show dramatic improvement in muscle strength, regaining facial expression, posture, and respiratory function within 1 min.

Marsh S, Pittard A. Neuromuscular disorders and anaesthesia. Part 2: Specific neuromuscular disorders. *Continuing Education in Anaesthesia Critical Care & Pain* 2011; 11 (4) 119–123.

17. D

Flush solution under pressure is required to maintain patency of an arterial line. There is no strong recommendation on the necessity of heparinized solution which can correctly be added or not depending on local protocols.

Blood sampling is common from arterial lines. When glucose is used as flush solution there may be resultant erroneously high glucose readings in blood sampling. There have been UK national alerts on severe hypoglycaemia from misdirected administration of insulin when glucose solutions are used to flush arterial lines. The Association of Anaesthetists of Great Britain and Ireland guidelines recommend saline 0.9% safe flush solution.

Membership of the Working Party: Woodcock TE, Cook TM, Gupta KJ, Hartle A. Arterial line blood sampling: preventing hypoglycaemic brain injury 2014. *Anaesthesia* 2014; 69: 380–385.

18. E

A tunnelled catheter requires additional expertise, is associated with reduced infection rates, and is more appropriate for long-term access i.e. months/years. The indication for central line placement in this patient (new septic episode) is likely to be of shorter duration so a non-tunnelled catheter is more appropriate. Multiple lumens are indicated. A left subclavian site would indicate a 24-cm device should be chosen for an adult.

Bodenham A, Babu S, Bennett J, et al. Association of Anaesthetists of Great Britain and Ireland: Safe vascular access 2016. *Anaesthesia* 2016; 71: 573–585.

19. D

It is important to read this question accurately. It does NOT ask for the best technique or the best anaesthetic or what is best for this particular patient. It asks about the best intubating conditions.

While many centres have moved away from the traditional thiopentone and suxamethonium rapid sequence induction technique, it continues to provide the best intubating conditions with or without the use of opioids. Of note, suxamethonium produces better intubation conditions when used with thiopentone when compared to its use with propofol.

Tran DTT, Newton EK, Mount VAH. Rocuronium vs. succinylcholine for rapid sequence intubation: A Cochrane systematic review. *Anaesthesia* 2017; 72: 765–777.

This review is an abridged version of a Cochrane review published in the Cochrane Database of Systematic Reviews (CDSR) 2015; 10: CD002788.

20. D

This is one of the few times where we would comply with the wishes of the relative over the patient. Ideally patients should make their wishes known to relatives to allow their agreement and authorization of the organ donation process. Despite the patient themselves having consented to this process, relatives can, and do, refuse permission.

Various strategies are being developed to reduce the number of families preventing organ donation in this way.

Death of a loved one is a traumatic time for relatives and no one would wish to increase their distress. Rather, building a relationship with relatives and explaining the process of donation and their relatives intentions to do so before he died is a more caring approach.

It is not necessary to discuss this with the coroner as there is a robust, ethical, and professional framework for doctors to work within.

Murphy P, Adams J. Ethico-legal aspects of organ donation. *Continuing Education in Anaesthesia Critical Care & Pain* 2013; 13 (4): 125–130.

Organ Donation NHS UK. Families saying no to donation results in missed transplant opportunities for UK patients. Available at: https://www.organdonation.nhs.uk/news-and-campaigns/news/families-saying-no-to-donation-results-in-missed-transplant-opportunities-for-uk-patients/

21. E

From the history, it can be assumed the patient spent a prolonged time in stages 2 and 3 of labour and delivery, in the lithotomy position. Such flexion of the thigh commonly causes compression and ischaemia of the lateral cutaneous nerve of thigh. This has no motor component and is known as meralgia paraesthetica. It accounts for up to one third of obstetric nerve palsies.

In the history there is no dermatomal distribution of symptoms therefore the symptoms are not due to nerve root pathology or disc prolapse. The fetal head can compress the lumbosacral trunk causing femoral and obturator nerve palsies and their associated typical symptoms (see reference). Postnatal obstetric palsies have an incidence of 1% and symptoms should be taken seriously.

Boyce H, Plaat F. Post-natal neurological problems. *Continuing Education in Anaesthesia Critical Care & Pain* 2013; 13 (2): 63–66.

22. A

The anaesthetic principle in this case is to use short-acting agents to allow rapid emergence and reduce the impact of anaesthetic agents on his OSA. Desflurane wears off most rapidly due to its insolubility (low blood/gas coefficient). Remifentanil has a half-life of approximately 3 min irrespective of the duration of the infusion (context specific half-life). Ventilation should be controlled with an endotracheal tube to maintain the airway. Spontaneous ventilation will not be adequate using a remifentanil infusion and the typical OSA patient is overweight with a large neck and a potentially difficult airway.

The patient also requires good analgesia with minimal use of opioids. An inguinal field block will provide this.

Regional anaesthesia would be a good option in this scenario for patients with normal INR. An INR of 1.5 precludes spinal anaesthesia.

Sedative premedication should be avoided and any CPAP support the patient uses at home should be available and continued in the postoperative period.

Care in a high dependency unit is usually indicated for these patients.

Guillermo Martinez, MD Peter Faber, Obstructive sleep apnoea. *Continuing Education in Anaesthesia Critical Care & Pain* 2011; 11 (1): 5–8.

23. B

Changing only the composition of the inspired gas mixture will take a long time at such a low FGF rate due to the inertia of the circle system. The quickest option to increase the end-tidal isoflurane concentration is to increase the FGF rate.

Nunn G. Low-flow anaesthesia, *Continuing Education in Anaesthesia Critical Care & Pain* 2008; 8 (1): 1–4.

24. B

The child's weight can be estimated to 22 or 23 kg with various commonly used formulae. The dose of morphine is 0.1–0.2 mg/kg which equates to a maximum of 4.6 mg morphine. Opioid related complications are the commonest cause of postoperative problems following tonsillectomy, particularly when sleep apnoea may be suspected. Though difficult to diagnose in children, a careful history must be taken as a diagnosis of OSA increases the rate of all cause post-operative complications from 1% up to 16–27%.

NSAIDs are routinely given. It is normal to have blood stained secretions post tonsillectomy and any problems the parents have are no contraindications to discharging the child.

Pearson A, Cook T. Litigation and complaints associated with day case anaesthesia. *BJA Education* 2017; 17 (9): 289–294.

Ravi R, Howell T. Anaesthesia for paediatric ear, nose, and throat surgery. *Continuing Education in Anaesthesia Critical Care & Pain* 2007 7 (2) 33–37.

25. A

Transdermal drug delivery occurs by diffusion down a concentration gradient from the patch to the skin. Low molecular weight, high potency, and high lipid solubility promote transdermal transfer of a drug.

A low melting point is desirable to promote release of the drug. The thickness of skin and fat is important as is the peripheral blood flow to the area. Metabolites have no effect on transdermal delivery of drug.

Bajaj S, Whiteman A, Brandner B. Transdermal drug delivery in pain management. *Continuing Education in Anaesthesia Critical Care & Pain* 2011 11 (2): 39–43.

26. C

A partial agonist binds to and activates a specific receptor, but has only partial efficacy when compared to a full agonist. Therefore the effect it can produce will always be sub-maximal, and less than a full agonist. Potency is the dose range over which a drug is active and partial agonists can higher or lower potency than the corresponding full agonist. A partial agonist, by definition, only binds to agonist receptors but can have antagonist effects, by occupying a proportion of receptors and preventing the full agonist reaching them, and so causes a net reduction in the response. Competitive antagonists compete for the same binding sites as the corresponding agonist whereas non-competitive antagonists have a separate binding site meaning their action cannot be overcome by increasing the dose of agonist.

Lambert DG. Drugs and receptors. *Continuing Education in Anaesthesia Critical Care & Pain* 2004; 4 (6): 181–184.

27. A

Bioavailability is increased as hepatic blood flow is reduced by up to 35% and less drug is extracted and lost to first pass metabolism.

Phase I reactions (reduction and oxidation) in the liver are greatly reduced, while phase 2 reactions (conjugation) are largely maintained. Cytochrome p450 genetic polymorphisms remain by far the most important cause of metabolic variability than ageing.

Drug metabolism by the liver may be flow dependent (most common) with a high extraction ratio or capacity dependent with a lower extraction ratio. Hepatic blood flow is reduced in the elderly and membrane transport mechanisms less efficient.

With increasing age the proportion of body fat increases relative to that of water and muscle mass which decrease. This means water soluble drugs will have a lower volume of distribution (VoD) and increased concentration in the extra cellular fluid. Fat soluble drugs have a higher VoD and a prolonged half life.

eGFR is significantly reduced in the elderly but this is due to co-existing disease (vascular disease, hypertension) rather than ageing per se.

Roberts F, Freshwater-Turner D. Pharmacokinetics and anaesthesia. *Continuing Education in Anaesthesia Critical Care & Pain* 2007 7 (1): 25–29.

Klotz U. Pharmacokinetics and drug metabolism in the elderly. *Drug Metabolism Reviews* 2009; 41(2): 67–76.

28. C

Normal fetal heart rate at term is 110–160 bpm and is frequently monitored on a CTG. The baseline is recorded as the mean heart rate over 10 min. A rate >160 bpm is classified as a fetal tachycardia and a rate <110 bpm is a fetal bradycardia. Variability refers to normal fluctuations in heart rate with normal variability being 5–25 bpm and is reassuring. It is measured from the peak to the trough heart rate of a CTG recording over a period of 1 min. A persistent absence of variability is considered a pre-terminal feature and carries with it a high probability of a hypoxic fetus.

Decelerations are transient reductions in fetal heart rate >15 bpm for at least 15 seconds. They can be early or late when observed against the timing of uterine contractions:

- Early decelerations are uniform in shape, mirror the contraction, and are a normal finding in labour. They are thought to be a result of fetal head compression during a contraction and should recover with relaxation of the uterus.
- Late decelerations are uniform and gradual in shape but they have a trough that occurs after the peak of a contraction. These are a possible sign of reduced fetal oxygenation

Accelerations are defined as a transient increase in fetal heart rate (>15 bpm for at least 15 seconds) and these tend to be associated with fetal activity. Although their presence is reassuring, absence in an otherwise normal CTG should not cause concern.

All the answers describe normal fetal heart rate. Both answers B and C show a concerning feature but the absence of variability indicates a higher concern for fetal hypoxia.

Jayasooriya G, Djapardy V. Intrapartum assessment of fetal well-being. *BJA Education* 2017; 17 (12): 406–411.

29. C

There are many specific criteria to be met for brainstem death testing or the diagnosis of death by neurological criteria. Although normocapnia is recommended in the general management of these patients in the Intensive Care Unit, in the specific incidence of performing apnoea testing the minute ventilation should be reduced to allow the $PaCO_2$ to rise to ≥6.0 kPa before commencing the test. At the end of the 5 min apnoea the recorded $PaCO_2$ should have risen ≥0.5 kPa. This is the case in both sets of tests. It has also been suggested that if the patient is a chronic retainer of CO_2 due to heavy smoking or chronic obstructive airway disease then it would be prudent to allow $PaCO_2$ to rise to ≥6.5 kPa prior to testing.

Form for diagnosis of death using neurological criteria. Available at: https://www.ficm.ac.uk/sites/default/files/Form%20for%20the%20Diagnosis%20of%20Death%20using%20Neurological%20Criteria%20-%20Full%20Version%20%282014%29.pdf

30. D

This patient has several risk factors for the development of hyperkalaemia including cardiac failure and likely use of angiotensin-converting enzyme inhibitors and diuretics, diabetes, and chronic renal impairment. A potassium level >7 mmol/L is classified as severe especially with ECG changes and urgent treatment is required.

The priority is to give calcium gluconate to stabilize the myocardium and then institute treatment to lower the serum potassium concentration such as insulin/dextrose infusion and nebulized salbutamol. You would stop drugs or infusions containing potassium. Haemodialysis may also be a definitive treatment.

The ECG changes associated with hyperkalaemia are tall tented T wave, flattening and loss of p waves, prolonged P-R interval, and widening of the QRS complex. Bradycardia and AV block are also common. These changes are progressive with increasing potassium concentrations and can eventually there will be ventricular fibrillation and cardiac arrest.

UK Renal Association. Clinical practice guidelines treatment of acute hyperkalaemia in adults. Available at: https://renal.org/wp-content/uploads/2017/06/hyperkalaemia-guideline-1.pdf

INDEX

Note: 'q' after the page number refers to questions, and 'a' to answers.

A

abdominal aortic aneurysm repair
  cross clamping 66q, 69q, 73a, 76a
  renal protection 69q, 76a
abdominal compartment syndrome 38q, 45a
ABO incompatibility 27a
accelerations, fetal heart rate 182a
acetyl cysteine therapy 150a
acid base disorders 145q, 151a
acoustic neuroma surgery, air embolism 109q, 115a
activated charcoal 150a
acupuncture 162–63a
  for back pain 116a
  for chronic headache
acute haemolytic transfusion reactions 27a
addiction 175a
adductor canal block 31a
adrenaline (epinephrine)
  in anaphylaxis 126a
  and cataract surgery 62a
  effect during cardiac arrest 40q, 47a
  in hypotension 29a
air embolism, intracranial surgery 109q, 115a
airway fires
  management 168q, 175–76a
  risk reduction 51q, 59a
airway management
  awake fibreoptic intubation 49q, 57a
  difficult intubation 42q, 48a, 49q, 57a
  dynamic airway assessment 52q, 59a
  for wisdom teeth extraction 53q, 60a
airway obstruction 35q, 43a
  children 119q, 124–25a, 127a
airway pressure changes 97q, 102a
airway pressure release ventilation 144q, 150a
albumin levels 17a
alcohol consumption, anaesthetic management 54q, 61a
alfentanil, patients with epilepsy 57a
allergic reactions 36q, 44a
  anaphylaxis 36q, 41q, 44a, 48a, 126a
alveolar gas equation 43a
Alzheimer's disease 5q, 12–13a, 83q, 92a
amiodarone, extravasation management 64q, 71a

amputation, chronic pain 156q, 160–61a
anaemia 11q, 18a, 82q, 90a
  indications for transfusion 22q, 29–30a
analgesia, postoperative 7q, 8q, 14a, 15a
  continuous wound infiltration 63q
  methadone users 11q, 18a
  oral regimens 65q, 72a
  tonsillectomy 53q, 60–61a
analysis of variance (ANOVA) 62a, 170q
anaphylaxis 36q, 44a, 126a
  potential causes 41q, 48a
ankle blocks 82q, 91a
anticoagulation
  citrate 145q, 151a
  and spinal anaesthesia 7q, 14a
antiemetics
  in Parkinson's disease 63q, 70a
  in QTc interval prolongation 51q, 58a
antiplatelet therapy, perioperative management 49q, 56, 56a,
    65q, 71a
  ticagrelor 81q, 89a
anxiety 32a
  children 83q, 91a
aortic cross clamping 66q, 73a
  clamp release 69q, 76a
  renal protection 69q, 76a
aortic stenosis 8q, 16a, 28a
  in pregnancy 169q, 177a
APACHE II 73a
Apfel score 87a
apnoea testing 174q, 182a
aprepitant 58a
arterial lines
  air bubbles in the system 41q, 48a
  damping 143q, 149a
  flush solution 171q, 179a
asthma 125–26a
  life-threatening features 39q, 46a
  pressure–volume curves 97q, 103a
atlanto-axial instability 33a
atrial fibrillation 28a
  risk assessment 66q, 73a
  rivaroxaban, perioperative management 67q, 73–74a

atrioventricular (AV) block 13a
autonomic dysreflexia 106q, 113a
awake craniotomy 109q, 115a
awake fibreoptic intubation 49q, 57a
awareness 71a

B

back pain 110q, 116a, 158q, 163–64a
Bell's palsy 57–58a
benign intracranial hypertension 132q, 139a
beta 2 transferrin assay 135a
betadine allergy 44a
bilirubin levels 17a
bioavailability, changes with age 181a
blackouts, history of 24q, 31–32a
blood cultures 29a
blood pressure measurement 93q, 98a
blood sugar, preoperative assessment 28a
blood transfusion
    indications for 22q, 29–30a
    Jehovah witnesses 22q, 29a
    oxyhaemoglobin dissociation curve 43a
    salvaged blood 130q, 131q, 136a, 138a
    transfusion reactions 19q, 27a
bone cement implantation syndrome 24q, 32a
botulinum toxin
    for chronic headache 162–63a
    for migraine 164a
botulism 154a
bradycardia, cardiac transplants 96q, 101a
brainstem death 146q
    apnoea testing 174q, 182a
    cardiovascular management 148q, 153a
    diabetes insipidus 152a
    organ donation 171q, 179a
breath stacking 70a
breathing difficulties
    children 120q, 121q, 125–26a, 127a
    postoperative 25q, 32a
Brief Pain Inventory 162a
bronchoscopes
    sterilization of 13a
    ventilating 119q, 125a
BTS CURB-65 149a
burns 41q, 48a

C

caesarean section
    aortic stenosis 169q, 177a
    intubating conditions 171q, 179a
    postoperative hypovolaemia 133q, 139–40a
capacity 58a
carbamazepine, in trigeminal neuralgia 159q, 164a
carbimazole 60a
carbon monoxide, oxyhaemoglobin dissociation curve 43a
carboxyhaemoglobin 33a
carcinoid tumours 8q, 16a

cardiac arrest
    adrenaline, therapeutic effect 40q, 47a
    airway management 35q, 43a
    circulatory access 40q, 47a
    hypothermia 37q, 44a
    neurological prognostication 36q, 44a
    posterior fossa surgery 106q, 112a
    ventricular fibrillation 40q, 47a
cardiac output measurement 93q, 98a
cardiac surgery, risk assessment 96q, 101a
cardiac transplants 96q, 101a
cardiogenic shock, intra-aortic balloon pumps 93q, 94q, 98a, 99a
cardiomyopathy, dilated 95q, 100a
cardiopulmonary exercise testing 82q, 83q, 90a, 91a
cardiorespiratory resuscitation see cardiac arrest
cardiotocography 173q, 182a
carotid endarterectomy 65q, 71a
cataract surgery
    antiplatelet therapy 49q, 56a
    and glaucoma 55q, 62a
caudal epidural steroid injection 116a
    adverse effects 157q, 162a
cell salvage 20q, 28a
central lines 171q, 179a
    catheter tip position checking 66q, 73a
    insertion in coagulopathy 146q, 151–52a
    ultrasound guidance 143q, 149a
cerebral salt wasting 152a
cerebrospinal fluid identification 129q, 135a
cervical spine abnormalities, rheumatoid arthritis 26q, 33a
cervical spine assessment 108q, 114a
chemosis 61a
child protection 117q, 123a
children see paediatrics
2-chloroprocaine 62a
choking 118q, 124a
cholinesterase deficiency 68q, 75a
chronic obstructive airway disease
    diagnosis 168q, 176a
    dynamic airway assessment 52q, 59a
    postoperative analgesia 65q, 72a
    severity grading 176–77a
    ventilatory management 64q, 70a
    weaning from ventilation 147q, 153a
chronic pain
    after amputation 156q, 160–61a
    back pain 110q, 116a, 158q, 163–64a
    caudal epidural steroid injection 157q, 162a
    headache 162–63a
after mastectomy 155q, 156q, 160a, 161a
    migraine 159q, 164a
    neuropathic pain 158q, 164a
    opioid-induced hyperalgesia 159q, 165a
    patient characteristics 157q, 162a
    post-herpetic neuralgia 158q, 163a
    serotonin syndrome 159q, 165a

in spinal cord injury 155q, 160a
transdermal drug administration 173q, 181a
trigeminal neuralgia 159q, 164a
chronic regional pain syndrome 155q, 160a
citrate anticoagulation 145q, 151a
coagulation testing 94q, 99a
coagulopathy, central line insertion 146q, 151–52a
codeine, variations in metabolism 60–61a
common peroneal nerve injury 27q, 138a
communication problems, non-English speakers 134q, 141–42a
community-acquired pneumonia
    infective pathogens 147q, 153a
    risk stratification 143q, 149a
compartment syndrome 33a
    abdominal 38q, 45a
competitive antagonists 181a
consent 29a
    children 83q, 91a, 119q, 125a
    lack of capacity 50q, 58a
    non-English speakers 134q, 141–42a
    for obstetric epidural anaesthesia 133q, 140a
    for organ donation 171q, 179a
    for postoperative analgesia 96q, 101–2a
continuous local anaesthetic wound infiltration 63q, 70a
coronary artery bypass grafts
    complications 169q, 177a
    risk assessment 96q, 101a
corticosteroids see steroids
cough suppression 50q, 57a
Creutzfeldt–Jacob disease 107q, 113a
croup 125–26a, 126
Cushing's disease 113a
cyanosis, ventricular septal defect 95q, 100a
cystic fibrosis 83q, 91a

D

damping, arterial lines 48a, 143q, 149a
data spread 167q, 175a
DC cardioversion, transthoracic electrical
        impedance 35q, 43a
D-dimers 45a
decelerations, fetal heart rate 182a
delirium, risk minimization 9q, 17a
dementia, pain assessment 157q, 161–62a
depth of anaesthesia
    increasing 172q, 180a
    monitoring 109q, 115a
dexamethasone, PONV prophylaxis 58a
diabetes
    perioperative management 79q, 87a
    preoperative assessment 28a
diabetes insipidus 152a
diabetic ketoacidosis 87a
difficult airways 42q, 48a, 49q, 57a
    awake fibreoptic intubation 49q, 57a
dilated cardiomyopathy 95q, 100a
donepezil, perioperative management 83q, 92a

Down's syndrome, consent issues 50q, 58a
droperidol 58a
drug distribution, changes with age 181a
drug interactions
    in Alzheimer's disease 12–13a
    in Parkinson's disease 15a
drug metabolism, changes with age 181a
Dupuytren's contracture excision, regional blocks 23q, 31a
dural puncture 133q
    CSF identification 129q, 135a
    headache risk reduction 130q, 136a, 137a
    management during labour 140a
    sixth nerve palsy 136a
dynamic airway assessment 52q, 59a

E

Eaton–Lambert syndrome 154a
echocardiography
    aortic stenosis 8q, 16a
    pulmonary thromboembolism 45a
ecstasy overdose 147q, 153a
Edmonton Frail Scale 86a
edrophonium challenge test 178a
ejection systolic murmurs 28a
elderly patients, pharmacokinetics 173q, 181–82a
electrocardiography (ECG)
    hyperkalaemia 183a
    myocardial infarction 6q, 13a
    progressive PR interval prolongation 6q, 13a
    prolonged QTc interval 51q, 58a
electroconvulsive therapy (ECT), adverse
        effects 79q, 86–87a
electroencephalography (EEG), neurological prognostication
        after cardiac arrest 44a
emergency surgery 68q, 75a
    consent issues 96q, 101–2a
endotracheal tube choice
    children 122q, 128a
    for pneumonectomy 97q, 102a
end-tidal oxygen fraction (FETO$_2$) 74a
enhanced recovery after surgery 14a
enteral feeding 147q, 153a, 170q, 178a
ephedrine 29a
epidural anaesthesia
    after amputation 161a
    complications 129q
    consent issues 133q, 140a
    CSF identification 129q, 135a
    dural puncture 130q, 133q, 136a, 137a, 140a
    postoperative 158q, 163a
    rivaroxaban, perioperative management 67q, 73–74a
epiglottitis 125–26a, 126
epilepsy
    driving regulations 108q, 114a
    use of opioids 50q, 57a
epinephrine see adrenaline
erythromycin, as a prokinetic 74a

etomidate, effect on intraocular pressure 54q, 61a
EURO Score II 96q, 101a
evidence levels 10q, 17a
extracorporeal membrane oxygenation 144q, 150–51a
extravasation management, amiodarone 64q, 71a
extubation 9q, 17a, 147q, 153a
    after mandibular advancement surgery 50q, 57a
exudates, Light's criteria 154a
eye injuries 54q, 61a
    anaesthetic induction agents 54q, 61a
eye surgery, regional analgesia, complications 53q, 61a

F

facet joint injections 116a
facial nerve stimulation 54q, 62a
facial weakness 57–58a
famciclovir 163a
femoral nerve block 31a
fentanyl patches 173q, 181a
ferritin levels 18a
fetal circulation 120q, 126a
fetal heart rate 173q, 182a
fluid therapy, children 121q
foot drop 19q, 27a
    postpartum 138a
fractured neck of femur 31a
    pain management 25q, 33a
    preoperative anaemia 22q, 29–30a
    preoperative assessment 20q, 24q, 28a, 31–32a,
        168q, 176a
    spinal anaesthesia 21q, 29a
    timing of surgery 31a
frailty indicators 78q, 86a

G

gabapentin
    in post-herpetic neuralgia 163a
    in trigeminal neuralgia 164a
gag suppression 50q, 57a
galantamine 5q
gastro-oesophageal reflux 68q, 75a
gastro-oesophageal variceal bleeding 74a
Glasgow Coma Scale, prognostication after cardiac
        arrest 44a
glaucoma 55q, 62a
goitre, preoperative assessment 53q, 60a
greater occipital nerve blocks 162–63a
Guillain–Barré syndrome 115a, 152a, 154a

H

HADS score 162a
haematemesis 67q, 74a
haemoglobin levels 18a
haemorrhage
    tranexamic acid 39q, 47a
    traumatic amputation 37q, 45a
head injury 38q, 46a

avoidance of secondary brain injury 105q, 111a
    brainstem death 146q, 152a
    clearing the cervical spine 108q, 114a
    fixed dilated pupil 110q
    imminent herniation 116a
headache
    chronic 157q, 162–63a
    migraine 159q, 164a
    post- dural puncture 130q, 133q, 136a, 137a, 140a
    postpartum 170q, 178a
heat loss 19q, 27a
heliox 59a
hip fracture see fractured neck of femur
Hospital Episode Statistics 73a
hyaluronidase, in extravasation management 71a
hydrocephalus, obstetric management 130q, 137a
hydrocortisone see steroids
hyperkalaemia 174q, 182–83a
hypermagnesaemia 139a
hypertension 80q, 88a
    postoperative analgesia 65q, 72a
hyperthermia, oxyhaemoglobin dissociation curve 43a
hypocalcaemia, post thyroidectomy 51q, 59a
hyponatraemia 10q, 18a, 152a
    ecstasy overdose 147q, 153a
hypopituitarism, post-partum 40q, 47a
hypotension
    after aortic cross clamp release 69q, 76a
    bone cement implantation syndrome 24q, 32a
    after caesarean section 133q, 139–40a
    cardiac transplants 96q, 101a
    after phaeochromocytoma resection 69q, 75–76a
    during posterior fossa surgery 109q, 115a
    during spinal anaesthesia 21q, 29a
    TURP syndrome 78q, 85a
hypothermia 37q, 44a
    preoperative 80q, 87–88a
hypoventilation, postoperative 68q, 75a

I

induction agents, effect on intraocular pressure 54q, 61a
infra-patellar nerve, adductor canal block 31a
insulin therapy, perioperative management 79q, 87a
intensive care
    acid base disorders 145q, 151a
    airway pressure release ventilation 144q, 150a
    arterial lines 143q, 149a, 171q, 179a
    brainstem death 146q, 148q, 152a, 153a, 171q,
        174q, 182a
    central line insertion 171q, 179a
    in coagulopathy 146q, 151–52a
    ultrasound guidance 143q, 149a
    citrate anticoagulation 145q, 151a
    ecstasy overdose 147q, 153a
    enteral feeding 147q, 153a, 178a
    extracorporeal membrane oxygenation 144q, 150–51a
    pain management 169q, 177a

paracetamol overdose 144q, 149–50a
pleural fluid biochemistry 148q, 154a
prone ventilation 145q, 151a
smoke inhalation 146q, 152a
weaning from ventilation 147q, 153a
interquartile range 175a
interscalene block 31a
phrenic nerve palsy 32a
intra-aortic balloon pumps
choice of gas 167q, 175a
contraindications 93q, 98a
side effects of insertion 94q, 99a
intraocular pressure, effect of induction agents 54q, 61a
intraosseous access 47a
intrathecal catheters, PDPH reduction 137a
intravenous drug use, causes of weakness 148q, 154a
intravenous fluids, children 121q, 127a
intubating conditions 171q, 179a
intubation
awake fibreoptic intubation 49q, 57a
difficult 42q, 48a, 49q, 57a
mouth opening limitation 54q, 61a
after thermal injury 48a
iodine, in thyrotoxicosis 60a
iron deficiency anaemia 11q, 18a, 82q, 90a
isolated forearm technique 72a
itch, after spinal anaesthesia 20q, 28a

K

ketamine
paediatric dose 125a
site of action 156q, 161a
knee arthroscopy, regional blocks 23q, 31a
Koivurata score 87a
Korotkov sounds 93q, 98a

L

laparoscopy, anaesthetic management 79q, 87a
laryngeal mask airways, paediatric 120q, 126–27a
laryngomalacia 125–26a
laryngospasm 24q, 32a, 71a, 118q, 124a
children 121q, 127a
laser airway surgery, airway fires 51q, 59a, 168q, 175–76a
lateral cutaneous nerve of the thigh 30a, 180a
latex allergy 44a
latissimus dorsi flaps, perfusion optimization 78q, 85a
Lee's revised cardiac risk index 73a
leg pain and swelling, differential diagnosis 25q, 33a
leucodepletion filters 136a, 138a
levodopa, perioperative management 7q, 15a
lidocaine
for cataract surgery 62a
topical administration 49q, 57a
lidocaine patches 163a
lidocaine spray 118q, 124a
Light's criteria 154a
lithotomy position, nerve injury 138a, 180a

liver, synthetic function assessment 9q, 17a
liver disease, risk assessment 80q, 82a
local anaesthetics
avoidance of intravenous injection 118q, 123–24a
continuous wound infiltration 63q, 70a
toxicity 23q, 30a, 39q, 46a
lung surgery
airway pressure changes 97q, 102a
endotracheal tube choice 97q, 102a
postoperative analgesia 96q, 101a
preoperative assessment 84a, 95q, 100–1a

M

magnetic resonance imaging, contraindications 106q, 112a
malignant hyperthermia 67q, 74a
mandibular advancement surgery, extubation 50q, 57a
mannitol 116a
indications for use 168q, 176a
Marsh model 76a
mastectomy, chronic pain 155q, 156q, 160a, 161a
meralgia paraesthetica 30a, 180a
metabolic acidosis 151a
metabolic alkalosis 39q, 46a
metaraminol 29a
methadone use, postoperative analgesia 11q, 18a
methaemoglobin, oxyhaemoglobin dissociation curve 43a
metoclopramide 58a
midazolam, paediatric dose 125a
migraine 159q, 164a
Minto model 76a
misoprostol, in postpartum haemorrhage 137a
mitral regurgitation 94q, 98–99a
Mobitz type 1 block 13a
Mobitz type 2 block 13a
mock exams 1
monitoring
for depth of anaesthesia 109q, 115a
minimum standards 5q, 12a
of neuromuscular blockade 65q, 71–72a
for venous air embolism 105q, 111a
morphine
conversion of IV to oral therapy 72a
paediatric doses 123a
for tonsillectomy pain 60–61a
motor neurone disease 115a
mouth opening limitation 54q, 61a
multiple sclerosis 81q, 89a, 115a
murmurs 28a, 168q, 176a
paediatric 118q, 124a
Murray score 150a
muscle relaxants see neuromuscular blockade
myasthenia gravis 108q, 114a, 115a, 154a, 170q, 178a
myocardial infarction
NSTEMI 37q, 45a
perioperative 5q, 6q, 12a, 13a
myocardial oxygen demand reduction 37q, 45a
myotonic dystrophy, neuromuscular blockade 66q, 72a

N

neck dissection, postoperative dyspnoea 52*q*, 60*a*
necrotizing fasciitis 21*q*, 29*a*
nefopam 165*a*
neostigmine, drug interactions 12–13*a*
nephrectomy, continuous local anaesthetic wound
    infiltration 63*q*, 70*a*
neuromuscular blockade
  anaphylactic reactions 48*a*
  cholinesterase deficiency 68*q*, 75*a*
  drug interactions 5*q*, 12–13*a*
  monitoring 65*q*, 71–72*a*
  in myotonic dystrophy 66*q*, 72*a*
  re-administration after routine reversal 75*a*
neuropathic pain 158*q*, 164*a*
  in spinal cord injury 160*a*
nitrous oxide 155*q*, 160*a*
non-accidental injury 117*q*, 123*a*
non-ST elevation myocardial infarction (NSTEMI) 37*q*, 45*a*
noradrenaline (norepinephrine)
  after phaeochromocytoma resection 75–76*a*
  use in hypotension 29*a*

O

obesity
  antenatal 134*q*, 141*a*
  postoperative hypoxaemia 68*q*, 75*a*
obstetrics
  aortic stenosis 169*q*, 177*a*
  benign intracranial hypertension 132*q*, 139*a*
  caesarean section
  aortic stenosis 169*q*, 177*a*
  intubating conditions 171*q*, 179*a*
  postoperative hypovolaemia 133*q*, 139–40*a*
  cardiotocography 173*q*, 182*a*
  causes of death 129*q*, 136*a*
  causes of haemorrhage 131*q*, 137*a*
  dural puncture 130*q*, 133*q*, 136*a*, 140*a*
  epidural requests 133*q*, 140*a*
  hydrocephalus 130*q*, 137*a*
  non-English speakers 134*q*, 141–42*a*
  obesity 134*q*, 141*a*
  postpartum haemorrhage 131*q*
  postpartum headache 129*q*, 136*a*, 170*q*, 178*a*
  postpartum hypotension 133*q*, 139–40*a*
  postpartum neurological deficit 129*a*, 131*q*, 136*a*, 138*a*,
    172*q*, 180*a*
  pre-eclampsia 132*q*, 139*a*
  salvaged blood transfusion 130*q*, 131*q*, 136*a*, 138*a*
  supraventricular tachycardia 133*q*, 141*a*
obstructive sleep apnoea (OSA) 6*q*, 13–14*a*, 80*q*, 88*a*,
  172*q*, 180*a*
obturator nerve palsy 138*a*
octreotide 16*a*
oculomotor nerve palsy 57–58*a*
ondansetron 58*a*
ophthalmic surgery, regional analgesia 53*q*, 61*a*

opioid addiction 175*a*
opioid dependence 167*q*, 174*q*, 175*a*
opioid-induced hyperalgesia 159*q*, 165*a*
opioid itching 28*a*
opioid tolerance 175*a*
opioids 14*a*
  for back pain 116*a*, 163*a*
  cough/gag suppression 57*a*
  and epilepsy 50*q*, 57*a*
  methadone 11*q*, 18*a*
  oral regimens 72*a*
  oxycodone 8*q*, 15*a*
  paediatric use 123*a*, 180–81*a*
organ donation, consent 171*q*, 179*a*
oxycarbamazine, in trigeminal neuralgia 164*a*
oxycodone 8*q*, 15*a*
oxygen, alveolar partial pressure 35*q*, 43*a*
oxyhaemoglobin dissociation curve 35*q*, 43*a*

P

pacemakers 15*a*
  coding 95*q*, 100*a*
  perioperative management 7*q*, 15*a*
paediatrics 116*a*
  airway obstruction 119*q*, 124–25*a*
  anaphylaxis 126*a*
  breathing difficulties 120*q*, 121*q*, 125–26*a*, 127*a*
  croup vs. epiglottitis 126
  choking 118*q*, 124*a*
  endotracheal tube choice 122*q*, 128*a*
  heart murmurs 118*q*, 124*a*
  intravenous fluids 121*q*, 127*a*
  laryngeal mask airways 120*q*, 126–27*a*
  laryngospasm 121*q*, 127*a*
  morphine dose 123*a*, 180–81*a*
  non-accidental injury 117*q*, 123*a*
  paracetamol doses 117*q*, 123*a*
  refusal of treatment 83*q*, 91*a*, 119*q*, 125*a*
  rising fractional inspired CO_2 117*q*, 123*a*
  sickle cell disease 119*q*, 125*a*, 127*a*
  upper respiratory tract infections 121*q*, 127*a*
  ventilating bronchoscopes 119*q*, 125*a*
  VSD correction 95*q*, 100*a*
  weight estimation 126–27*a*
pain assessment 157*q*, 162*a*
  in dementia 157*q*, 161–62*a*
pain management
  fractured neck of femur 25*q*, 33*a*
  in intensive care 169*q*, 177*a*
  rib fractures 23*q*, 30*a*
  see *also* back pain; chronic pain; headache; postoperative
    analgesia
pain physiotherapy 163*a*
paired t-test 62*a*
paracetamol
  overdose 144*q*, 149–50*a*
  paediatric doses 117*q*, 123*a*

paraesthesia, causes 109q, 115a
paravertebral block
    complications 93q, 98a
    indications 167q, 175a
Parkinson's disease
    antiemetics 63q, 70a
    perioperative management 7q, 15a
parotidectomy 54q, 62a
partial agonists 173q, 181a
pass rate 1
peripheral nerve injuries 63q, 70a
    common peroneal nerve 27a
    lateral cutaneous nerve of the thigh 30a
peripheral nerve stimulation, neuromuscular blockade
        monitoring 71a
    phaeochromocytoma 69q, 75–76a
phantom limb pain 156q, 160–61a
pharmacokinetics, changes with age 173q, 181–82a
phenelzine 29a
phenoxybenzamine 75–76a
phentolamine, in extravasation management 71a
phenylephrine 29a
phenytoin, in trigeminal neuralgia 164a
phrenic nerve palsy 32a
pilocarpine 62a
pituitary, Sheehan's syndrome 40q, 47a
pituitary adenoma 107q, 113a
placebo effect 156q, 161a
pleural fluid biochemistry 148q, 154a
pneumonectomy
    airway pressure changes 97q, 102a
    endotracheal tube choice 97q, 102a
    preoperative assessment 77q, 84a
pneumonia
    community-acquired 143q, 149a
    infective pathogens 147q, 153a
Pneumonia Severity Score Index 149a
pneumothorax 97q, 102a
positive predictive value 68q, 74a
posterior fossa surgery
    air embolism 109q, 115a
    cardiac arrest 106q, 112a
    operative positions 108q, 114a
    venous air embolism detection 105q, 111a
posterior myocardial infarction 13a
post-herpetic neuralgia 158q, 163a
postoperative analgesia 7q, 8q, 14a, 15a
    amputation 160–61a
    consent 96q, 101–2a
    continuous wound infiltration 63q, 70a
    lung surgery 96q, 101a
    mastectomy 161a
    methadone users 11q, 18a
    oral regimens 65q, 72a
    thoracic epidural 158q, 163a
    tonsillectomy 53q, 60–61a

postoperative myocardial infarction 6q, 13a
postoperative nausea and vomiting (PONV)
    prophylaxis in QTc interval prolongation 51q, 58a
    risk prediction 79q, 87a
postpartum haemorrhage 137–38a
    causes 131q, 137a
    management 131q, 137a
postpartum headache 170q, 178a
postpartum hypotension 133q, 139–40a
postpartum neurological deficit 131q, 138a, 172q, 180a
P-POSSUM 73a
prednisolone see steroids
pre-eclampsia 132q, 139a
pregnancy 20q, 27–28a
    see also obstetrics
pregnancy-related death, causes 129q
preoperative assessment 20q, 28a, 78q
    AAGBI Safety Guideline 86a
    cardiopulmonary exercise testing 82q, 90a, 91a
    in cystic fibrosis 83q, 91a
    ECG abnormalities 6q, 13a
    EURO Score II 96q, 101a
    fractured neck of femur 168q, 176a
    frailty indicators 78q, 86a
    in goitre 53q, 60a
    hyperkalaemia 174q, 182–83a
    hypertension 80q, 88a
    iron deficiency anaemia 82q, 90a
    lung surgery 77q, 84a, 95q, 100–1a
    NICE guidance 86a
    obstructive sleep apnoea 6q, 88a, 172q, 180a
    pulmonary function tests 77q, 85a, 168q,
        176–77a
preoxygenation 67q, 74a
pressure–volume curves 97q, 103a
prone ventilation 145q, 151a
propofol
    effect on intraocular pressure 54q, 61a
    target-controlled infusion 69q, 76a
propranolol
    migraine prophylaxis 164a
    in thyrotoxicosis, mechanism of action 52q, 59a
propylthiouracil 60a
PROSEVA trial 151a
prothrombin time 17a
pulmonary artery catheters (PACs) 98a
pulmonary function tests 77q, 85a, 168q, 176–77a
    prior to lung surgery 77q, 84a, 95q, 100–1a
pulmonary lobectomy, preoperative assessment 77q, 84a,
        95q, 100–1a
pulmonary thromboembolism (PTE) 38q, 45a
pyloric stenosis 46a
pyrexia, malignant hyperthermia 67q, 74a

Q
QTc interval prolongation 51q, 58a

R

radial nerve block 21q, 29a
rapid sequence induction (RSI) 75a
   preoxygenation 67q, 74a
   after thermal injury 48a
receptor theory, partial agonists 173q, 181a
recombinant factor VIIa 137a
refeeding syndrome 147q, 153a, 170q, 178a
refusal of treatment, children 83q, 91a, 119q, 125a
regional blocks
   ankle block 82q, 91a
   for Dupuytren's contracture excision 23q, 31a
   interscalene block 31a, 32a
   for knee arthroscopy 23q, 31a
   local anaesthetic toxicity 23q, 30a, 39q, 46a
   in multiple sclerosis 89a
   for ophthalmic surgery 53q, 61a
   paravertebral block 93q, 98a, 167q, 175a
   radial nerve block 21q, 29a
remifentanil, cough/gag suppression 57a
renal protection, abdominal aortic aneurysm repair 69q, 76a
renal replacement lines 169q, 177a
respiratory failure
   airway pressure release ventilation 144q, 150a
   extracorporeal membrane oxygenation 144q, 150–51a
rheumatoid arthritis, cervical spine abnormalities 26q, 33a
rib fractures, pain management 23q, 30a
risk assessment 66q, 73a
   community-acquired pneumonia 143q, 149a
   EURO Score II 96q, 101a
rivaroxaban 7q, 14a
   perioperative management 67q, 73–74a
rocuronium 12–13a
   cholinesterase deficiency 75a
   re-administration after routine reversal 75a
ropinirole 7q, 15a, 63q, 70a
rotational thromboelastometry (ROTEM) 99a

S

salvaged blood transfusion 131q, 138a
   complications 130q, 136a
saphenous nerve, adductor canal block 31a
SBA questions
   fairness 1
   as a study aid 1–2
   subject matter 1
   subtleties 2
SBA technique 2
sedation, children 125a
seizures, driving regulations 108q, 114a
serotonin syndrome 159q, 165a
Sheehan's syndrome 40q, 47a
   pulmonary thromboembolism 45a
SIADH 152a
sickle cell disease 127a
   diagnosis 119q, 125a
   oxyhaemoglobin dissociation curve 43a

sixth nerve palsy 136a
skewed data 167q, 175a
SMART-COP 149a
smoke inhalation 146q, 152a
smoking cessation, early effects 26q, 33a
spinal anaesthesia
   anticoagulation management 7q, 14a
   hypotension 21q, 29a
   postoperative itching 20q, 28a
   during pregnancy 27–28a
spinal cord injuries
   anaesthetic requirements 105q, 111a
   autonomic dysreflexia 106q, 113a
   chronic pain 155q, 160a
squint 50q, 57–58a
statistics 55q, 62a, 178a
   analysis of variance (ANOVA) 170q
   data spread 167q, 175a
   positive predictive value 68q, 74a
stellate ganglion block, in extravasation management 71a
stents, cardiac 81q, 89a
sterilization processes 6q, 13a
   contamination risk 10q, 17a
sterilized devices, labelling 9q, 17a
steroids
   in extravasation management 71a
   perioperative management 8q, 16a
STOP-BANG criteria 13–14a, 88a
stridor 64q, 71a
   children 120q, 125–26a
   after thyroidectomy 51q, 58–59a
stump pain 156q, 160–61a
subarachnoid haemorrhage
   complications 107q, 113a
   grading 106q, 111–12a, 112
subglottic airways 52q, 59a
succinylcholine
   cholinesterase deficiency 75a
   after thermal injury 48a
supraclavicular block 31a
supraglottic airways 52q, 59a
supraventricular tachycardia, in pregnancy 133q, 141a
suxamethonium, drug interactions 12–13a
syndrome of inappropriate ADH production (SIADH) 18a

T

target-controlled infusions (TCIs), propofol 69q, 76a
Tecfidera (dimethyl fumarate) 81q, 89a
Tensilon challenge test 178a
terlipressin 74a
thiamine, enteral feeding 178a
thigh pain 22q, 30a
thiopental, effect on intraocular pressure 54q, 61a
thoracic outlet syndrome 65q, 72a
thoracic trauma 94q, 99a
thoracotomy, postoperative analgesia 96q, 101a
thrombocytopaenia, central line insertion 146q, 151–52a

thromboelastography 94*q*, 99*a*
thromboprophylaxis 49*q*, 56*a*
thyroidectomy
    postoperative hypocalcaemia 51*q*, 59*a*
    postoperative stridor 51*q*, 58–59*a*
    preoperative assessment 53*q*, 60*a*
thyrotoxicosis
    antithyroid drugs 60*a*
    propranolol, mechanism of action 52*q*, 59*a*
ticagrelor, perioperative management 81*q*, 89*a*
tongue studs 82*q*, 90*a*
tonsillectomy
    airway obstruction 119*q*, 124–25*a*
    laryngospasm 118*q*, 124*a*
    postoperative analgesia 53*q*, 60–61*a*
    postoperative discharge 172*q*, 180–81*a*
tooth avulsion 10*q*, 18*a*
topiramate 164*a*
total intravenous anaesthesia (TIVA) 69*q*, 76*a*
tracheostomy
    airway obstruction 35*q*, 43*a*
    postoperative dyspnoea 52*q*, 60*a*
train of four (TOF) monitoring 72*a*
tranexamic acid 39*q*, 47*a*
    in postpartum haemorrhage 137*a*
transdermal drug administration 173*q*, 181*a*
transfusion reactions 19*q*, 27*a*
    salvaged blood 130*q*, 136*a*
translation services 141–42*a*
transthoracic electrical impedance 35*q*, 43*a*
transurethral resection of the prostate 78*q*
    TURP syndrome 85*a*
traumatic amputation 37*q*, 45*a*

trigeminal neuralgia 159*q*, 164*a*
t-test 62*a*

U
ulnar nerve injuries 70*a*
ultrasound guidance, nerve blocks 21*q*, 29*a*
ultrasound probes 143*q*, 149*a*
upper gastrointestinal bleeding (UGIB) 67*q*, 74*a*
upper respiratory tract infections 81*q*, 89*a*
    children 121*q*, 127*a*
urea and electrolytes, preoperative assessment 28*a*

V
vasopressin, after phaeochromocytoma resection 75–76*a*
vecuronium, re-administration after routine reversal 75*a*
venous air embolism 105*q*, 111*a*
ventilating bronchoscopes 119*q*, 125*a*
ventilatory management, COPD 64*q*, 70*a*
ventricular fibrillation 40*q*, 47*a*
ventricular septal defect (VSD) correction 95*q*, 100*a*
viral encephalitis 154*a*
viscoelectric point-of-care devices 94*q*, 99*a*
vitamin K 137*a*

W
warming 80*q*, 87–88*a*
weakness, causes 146*q*, 148*q*, 152*a*, 154*a*, 170*q*, 178*a*
weaning from ventilation 147*q*, 153*a*
weight estimation, children 126–27*a*
Wenckebach phenomenon 13*a*
Wilcoxon signed rank test 62*a*
wisdom teeth extraction, airway management 53*q*, 60*a*
work of breathing 97*q*